*An amusing history
of American medicine*

THE HUMOR
OF HEALING

Dr. Donald A. Johnson

Badger Books Inc.
Oregon, Wis.

ISBN (10) 1-932542-13-2
ISBN (13) 9781932542134

Badger Books Inc./Waubesa Press
P.O. Box 192
Oregon, WI 53575
Toll-free phone: (800) 928-2372
Fax: (608) 835-3638
Email: books@badgerbooks.com
Web site: www.badgerbooks.com
Library of Congress Cataloging-in-Publication Data
Johnson, Donald A., MD.
  The humor of healing : an amusing history of American medi-
cine / Donald A.
Johnson.
    p. ; cm.
  Includes index.
  ISBN 1-932542-13-2 (alk. paper)
  1. Medicine--United States--Anecdotes. 2. Medicine--United
States--History--Anecdotes.
  [DNLM: 1. Medicine. 2. Wit and Humor--history.] I. Title.

R705.J64 2005
610'.2'07--dc22
                                   2005000055

Contents

1.
The Humor of Healing

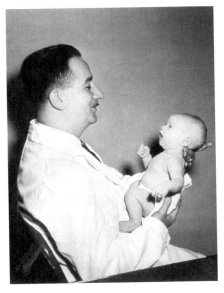

Is there humor in sickness and disability? Illness is alarming; it is a trying, somber experience for those who are sick and disabled and for the doctors who care for them.

But humor is an element of human nature; it bursts forth even in the most tragic circumstances.

Life is compounded of laughter and tears and inasmuch as the medical arena provides the best theater of life, it follows that humor has a large role in the dramas that play there.

A sense of humor is generally regarded as a desirable trait in a doctor. Those who are ill appreciate being cheered up. They need to be cheered up. Surely a doctor who dispirited his patients would be intolerable.

And doctors need a sense of humor; they needs relief from the anxiety that is their daily fare. Doctors' duties involve them in a mixture of tragedy and comedy; they are called upon to weep with those who weep and laugh with those who laugh. The humorous and the pathetic are often found side by side. A doctor is fortunate if the stress of his work is lightened by a hearty sense of humor.

A sick person is equally fortunate if he or she has a sense of humor. Many experiences can be seen as either tragic or comical depending on one's mood or point of view. In times of trial, humor sustains hope and tranquility; it encourages the acceptance of life as it is — contrasted to illusions of what it ought to be, while rejecting resignation. Humor projects a spirited resistance to the buffets of adversity.

An eighty-year-old man, troubled by a loss of memory, described his distress and exhibited his spirit in a note to his doctor:

I'm becoming more forgetful. And it worries me a bit.

Is this just normal aging? Or is there more than that to it? In the morning I may wonder: Did I brush my teeth or not? I feel the toothbrush. Is it wet? If it isn't, I forgot.

I'll put a bread roll in the oven. And when it bums, I'll recall I've thought of eggs and fruit and cheese. But I haven't eaten anything at all.

I'll think of something I should do. Perhaps it's up the stairs. But when I go up, I can't remember what it was or where?

I've given up my daily walks. All the streets seem new. Within a few blocks of home, I've gotten lost a time or two.

Forgetfulness is a trial. How much is normal? Who can say?

Yesterday, I thought of something I should do today. And today, I remembered it! Hooray!

An elderly man with Parkinson's disease had developed a

distressing tremor in his arms, but he discovered a positive aspect of his problem. He told his doctor that his success at fishing had increased significantly; the tremor gave just the right wiggle to his pole and line to attract the fish.

Humor is of ineffable value in medical relationships. Dr. William Wishard, a small-town practitioner in central Indiana, was once called to see a child who had an extensive skin infection on her face. The mother had covered her daughter's face with goose grease. Dr. Wishard advised removing the grease promptly; it encouraged the spread of the infection. Severe scarring of the child's face might result. But goose grease was a widely used and highly regarded folk remedy for skin disorders, and the mother declined to remove it.

Dr. Wishard's sense of humor dissolved the impasse smoothly. He asked if the grease came from a goose or from a gander. As he expected, the mother did not know. Then he asked if she knew the day of the month on which the bird had been killed. Of course, she did not. The doctor explained that without certainty on these two important points, it was unlikely that the goose grease was effective, and the mother, embarrassed by her apparent lack of knowledge, agreed to remove the grease immediately. Careful cleansing of the child's face soon brought evidence of healing.

Humor quells embarrassment. It can season the distasteful and rescue lapses and failures. When tragedy must be endured, humor can sometimes lighten the burden by transforming it into tragi-comedy.

On one such occasion, a young physician was examining a woman with lung cancer. The tumor had been removed surgically and radiation therapy had been directed to the lung to prevent recurrence. Had the treatment succeeded or failed? The physician put his stethoscope to the woman's chest hoping to hear normal breathing sounds over the affected part of the lung.

He was dismayed. He listened carefully and shifted his stethoscope several times, but there were no normal breathing sounds. The cancer had recurred and the treatments had failed. The doctor uttered an expletive almost under his breath. Then he blushed and hesitated. His patient surely had heard him. How to recover?

"That's OK," the lady said, "It's nice to know that you care."

Humor signals camaraderie, a sharing of difficulties that relaxes concern and fosters equanimity. It resolves troublesome situations that might otherwise disrupt fragile medical relationships.

Dr. Charles W. Mayo described a difficulty that arose when he joined the staff of the Mayo Clinic founded by his father and his uncle, Dr. William J. Mayo, both of whom were then retired. The young doctor was a very youthful looking man. He was thirty-three, but he looked like an adolescent. He was now *the* Dr. Mayo, but when he spoke of surgery, his youthful appearance aroused alarm and patients asked for another surgeon.

Dr. Mayo was a man of notably good humor. He examined a woman with gall bladder disease and advised her that she needed an operation. She accepted his recommendation and experienced the common mounting misgivings. When she asked who would do the surgery, her apprehension was obvious. Dr. Mayo's sense of humor resolved their mutual problem: "Dr. Judd has done thousands of operations on the gall bladder," he said earnestly. (Dr. E. Starr Judd had succeeded Dr. William Mayo as the principal surgeon at the Mayo Clinic.) "You may have him, or you may have me," Dr. Mayo continued, "I'm just starting and I can't afford to lose a patient."

"She grinned," he said, "and decided to have me do the operation."

What is a sense of humor? Books have been filled on the subject; it eludes comprehensive description. It falls into the category of things characterized by wags as, "I don't know what it is, but I know it when I see it." It's an attitude toward life. In medicine its essence is kindliness.

Students, nurses and doctors mobilize their sense of humor as they learn their roles. Then they use it to fulfill their duties. Those who are ill mobilize their sense of humor to cope with adversity. The anecdotes related here portray the humor of healing in America from the time of the early settlements to the present day. It is a panorama of the resilience and resourcefulness of the human spirit leavened by the foibles of the human situation. Insight into this pageant is the great reward of a medical practitioner's life.

It is elevating and it is amusing; it is a boon to the doctor's sense of humor. It begins with the curious circumstances that lead one to become a doctor.

2.
Why Be a Doctor?

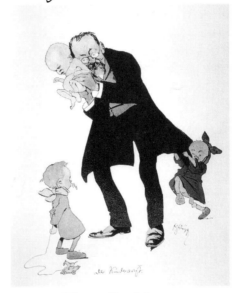

The pediatrician

It is widely believed that those who elect to become physicians are motivated by altruism, a wish to do good, or by visions of affluence. The reasons real doctors listed are more interesting.

"It was my mother," one physician recalled. When he was born, an intern held him up by the feet for his mother's viewing and prophesied: "This boy will some day be a fine doctor." The physician said, "Mother never forgot this incident, and she insisted that the prediction be fulfilled."

Mothers are powerful recruiters for the medical profession.

Another physician wrote: "My mother wasn't Jewish, but she was what you might call a Jewish Mother type, in that I was destined to be a doctor before I was born. She thought that was the kind of son she should have. And she brainwashed me so thoroughly that I never thought of being anything but a doctor."

Dr. Arthur Hertzler, the Kansas "Horse and Buggy Doctor," told how his mother's illness inspired him to become a doctor. His father switched from the Mennonite faith to Methodism without consulting his wife. Thereafter she was always sick on Sundays: too ill to attend church. Young Arthur overheard the doctor say that no treatment nor any amount of money would cure his mother of her trouble. This pronouncement stirred Arthur Hertzler to pursue a career in medicine to discover what illness it was that afflicted his mother and that money could not cure.

In early America, churchmen were held in much higher regard and fared far better financially than doctors. Ambitious young men were likely to aspire to the ministry. Some were diverted to medicine by unexpected developments. Gershom Bulkeley was a renowned healer in Connecticut between 1677 and 1713. Bulkeley was a clergyman, but his voice gave out and he could not preach. So, he became a physician instead. No qualifications were required at that time, only the need to earn a living and a desire to be a healer. Bulkeley gained great fame in Connecticut for his skill at healing.

In Massachusetts John Parks had planned to become a clergyman, but he had been raised in Calvinism and he had come to doubt its tenets. He struggled with his soul and decided that he could not conscientiously preach Calvinism — so he took to medicine instead.

Benjamin Rush was the first great doctor in America. He was a signer of the Declaration of Independence and he was the colonial medical authority. Rush graduated from Jersey College (later Princeton) in 1760 and decided to become a lawyer. Before returning to his home in Philadelphia he visited a boarding school in Maryland where he had been a student for five years before entering college. His boarding school teacher, a clergyman, advised him to study medicine and suggested a day of fasting followed by prayer; God would direct his choice. Rush wrote: "I am sorry to say I neglected the latter part of this excellent advice, but yielded to the former." And he added, "On what slight circumstances do our destinies in life seem to depend."

When the American frontier was moving westward, Daniel Drake was growing up in a log cabin in the wilderness of Kentucky. His father was a small-farm frontiersman working hard to derive a marginal subsistence from the land. His father's dream was that Daniel would be a doctor — a gentleman — in the image of one he had met and made friends with when he traveled west. Doctors were regarded as gentlemen, and a gentleman's status carried a prestige of its own unrelated to affluence.

In this era most American doctors were trained in an apprentice system. In 1800, when Daniel was fifteen, his father apprenticed him to a doctor in Cincinnati. Daniel was dismayed when he was informed of the plan. He thought he would like to become a tradesman; he had selected a saddle maker to whom he hoped to indenture himself in order to learn the trade.

Despite his disinclination, Daniel Drake became a physician. And then he became one of the giants of American medicine in the first half of the nineteenth century. He became a medical investigator, a medical writer, a teacher, a founder of medical schools, and a crusader for a better medical profession — all because his father traveled briefly with a physician on his way west.

In 1832, Dr. Daniel Drake described how most boys became doctors: "A neighboring physician wants a student to reside in his office. One son of the family is thought too weakly to labor on the farm.... too stupid for the Bar, and too immoral for the pulpit; the parents wish to have a gentleman in the family, and a doctor is a gentleman."

In this period, particularly on the western frontier, some young men drifted into healing and a few were even drafted. Priddy Meeks was a farmer in Illinois in 1815; he was an actively compassionate young man who acquired a knowledge of folk remedies and offered to share them with his neighbors: "Here when the sickly season of the year came on I visited many of the sick and was very successful in relieving them with roots and herbs, so much so that the community insisted I should quit work and go to doctoring. Such an idea had never entered my mind."

But he did go to doctoring. Then he joined the Mormons in Illinois and trekked west with them in 1846. Dr. Priddy Meeks (self taught and drafted) practiced medicine among the Mormons for more than forty years and to considerable acclaim.

In the South in 1833 Marion Sims graduated from college at Columbia, South Carolina. A southern boy who completed college and did not take a profession was regarded as a failure. Marion Sims felt that he was unsuited for the law, and he had no inclination toward the church. "There was nothing left for me to do," he wrote, "but to be a doctor — to study medicine or to disgrace my family."

His decision plunged his father into despair: "It is a profession for which I have the utmost contempt," his father wailed. "There is no science in it. There is no honor be achieved in it; no reputation to be made, and to think that my son should be going from house to house through this country, with a box of pills in one hand and a squirt can (enema pump) in the other... is a thought I never supposed I should have to contemplate."

Mr. Sims' appraisal of the medical profession was widely shared and was not too far from the mark,

Nonetheless Marion Sims became a surgeon. He devised an ingenious operation that put an end to a common complication of pregnancy that had shattered women's lives since creation. He created the specialty of gynecology. He founded the Woman's Hospital in New York, the first hospital of it's kind.

He demonstrated his surgical techniques in all of the capitals of Europe and was honored around the world.

He became one of the most eminent men in the history of American surgery.

Fathers with a greater insight into medicine were not better judges of their offspring. Dr. John Mitchell was a prominent physician in Philadelphia, a professor at the Jefferson Medical College. His son Silas seemed unmotivated: he was a dreamer — not an apt student. Dr. Mitchell urged his son to go into business; he was distressed when, in 1848, his son elected to study medicine. "You are wanting in nearly all of the qualities that go to make a success in medicine," he said.

But Silas had made his choice. He graduated from Jefferson Medical College in 1850. Dr. Silas Weir Mitchell became a founder of American neurology, a pioneer psychiatrist and the most eminent American authority in these fields during the Civil War era.

Among the fathers who tried to direct their offspring away from medicine, Dr. Adolf Gundersen set a record. Dr. Gundersen practiced in La Crosse, Wisconsin; he had seven sons. "I told them not to be doctors," he said, "I warned them against it, but they wouldn't listen to me." Six sons became physicians.

Of course dissuasion was not limited to doctors advising their sons. A young woman doctor recalled that her parents, her teachers, her counselors and her friends all thought that she was incapable of becoming a physician. This made her determined to do it — and she did.

Likewise, a college student debating the merits of dentistry and athletic coaching as careers, read the book *Arrowsmith,* and it persuaded him to add medicine to his considerations. He sought counseling from his dean of student affairs who advised him to drop medicine. "You don't have enough money," he was told. The student chose medicine and completed a medical education. "I resented his advice so I decided to go ahead," he said. He became an internationally renowned ophthalmologist.

Family tradition may exert a powerful influence directing one toward a life in medicine. Dr. John Black, a Pennsylvanian, seems to have had no choice in selecting his life's work. He entered the medical school of the University of Pennsylvania in 1800. His father was a doctor and his grandfather had been a doctor. "For this reason it was decreed by my family that I, willing or unwilling, should also become a physician."

In Hancock, New Hampshire, in the late 1800s, John Coolidge became a physician in a reaction against fate. He operated a farm and a grist mill. He had a son who died three days after his birth. Later a daughter died, also three days after birth, and then his wife died from complications associated with the daughter's birth. John Coolidge was aroused: these deaths were not necessary; he would do something about it. He sold his farm and grist mill and enrolled in Dartmouth College to study medicine.

In the same era a Wisconsin farm boy saw his future in a vision that was almost magical. He was working in a field of oats on an unbearably hot day when a buggy with a white canvas top appeared on a road shaded by a few maple trees at one end of the field. The buggy was drawn by a horse with a white fly net covering its entire body and carried a well-known doctor dressed in a white linen suit.

The buggy drifted along in the cool shade and seemed to the boy in the hot field like a "scene from paradise." He dropped his rake and watched the idyllic spectacle until the buggy passed leisurely out of sight, at which moment his future was revealed and decided: "Yes," he exulted, "I will be a doctor. Why haven't I thought of it before?" Franklin Martin graduated the Chicago Medical College in 1880. He became a surgeon of international repute, founder of a prestigious medical journal and was instrumental in the creation of a great society of surgeons devoted to the improvement of surgery.

The motivations to study medicine became more diverse as the country developed and the profession expanded. The father of James Fisher created a cattle ranch in Illinois during the 1870s and subsequently established his own packing house in Chicago. He encouraged his son to study veterinary medicine, which would fit him to take charge of and advance the enterprise. James Fisher enrolled in the Harvard School of Veterinary Medicine in 1891.

In Boston he met a young lady of social prominence who became the focus of his thoughts. He described her as being so prominent that she spoke to the Cabots and to the Lowells and to God. But when she spoke to James she "made it quite emphatic that she would never marry a horse doctor."

"Upon cross-examination," James Fisher discovered that she might look favorably on a medical degree so he transferred to the Harvard Medical School and graduated a doctor. Then he became a psychiatrist, focused his thoughts on a different young woman and married her.

James Fisher's path to a career in medicine is one that would never be traced in the absence of an autobiographical sketch. Undoubtedly there are many inscrutable motivations.

Jesters have proposed some that probably have a kernel of truth: the pediatrician who wanted to encourage better mothering than his mother had provided for him, the obstetrician who was intent on finding out more about where he came from, and the psychiatrist whose top priority was to save himself.

But there are autobiographical accounts that are equally amusing. One physician recalled how he worked in the local post office as a boy and began to read a doctor's copy of a medical journal that came through the mail unwrapped. Then, when their paths crossed, he began to ask the doctor questions. Then he assisted the doctor in his office and from there he went to medical school.

And the second female to graduate from the medical school of the University of Oregon told how as a young girl she watched a very attractive young woman walk by her home each morning. When she learned that the woman was a medical student walking to school, she thought, "If that's what women doctors look like, I want to be one."

For William Carlos Williams, the "Poet of Paterson" (New Jersey), the motive for becoming a physician was the unlikely one of gaining leisure. He said that he chose medicine so that he would have time to write. And a young contemporary in Minneapolis sought tranquility. He had directed his college studies toward law, but he "recognized the meanness in human beings which so often reveals itself in disputes over property and over injustices, real and imagined, and I was doubtful about devoting myself to such things for a lifetime." He became a doctor instead. Leisure and tranquility in medicine?

Boys growing up on progressive Midwestern farms in the early 1900s were immersed in botany and biology, elements of medicine, without knowing it; it was a grand basis for a medical career. Owen Wangensteen grew up on a farm in Minnesota and loved it; he was delighted by the animals and intrigued by the marvelous growth of the crops.

His father acquired fifty specially bred sows to upgrade the quality of his hogs and was dismayed to discover, when the time came, that the breeding process had produced sows that were unable to deliver their young. A veterinarian was called, but he was unable to bring about the delivery of the piglets. He advised shipping the hogs to market immediately; sell them before they die.

Owen Wangensteen searched through all of the available farm magazines for a solution; a considerable family investment was at stake. He acquired an advertised snare device that was said to be helpful: one could snare the piglets and pull them out — but it did not work.

In the course of experimenting with the snares Owen Wangensteen discovered that the best instrument was his hand. He lost two sows while learning to be a porcine obstetrician, but he delivered the other forty-eight hogs and saved most of the piglets. He was absent from school for three weeks to accomplish it.

When this experience was completed, "my father would hear of nothing, but that I should become a doctor." But Owen Wangensteen liked the farm. He sought a compromise and suggested to his father that he become a veterinarian. He could practice the veterinary science and continue to be a farmer. He went off to college and discussed the matter with his father each summer while caring for the animals and pitching hay.

After completing three years of college he "capitulated to my father's wishes" and entered medical school. He became a professor and chief of surgery at the University of Minnesota School of Medicine, an illustrious teacher and medical investigator and a leader in the medical affairs of the University of Minnesota for more than a quarter of a century (1930-1967).

It is clear that many young people become doctors as a result of events or circumstances that are unlikely to ever be repeated. This was surely the case of one contemporary physician who set out to be a chemical engineer and pursued that end contentedly until one night at dinner with his girlfriend. He reeked of hydrogen sulfide which smells like rotten eggs; the fumes had penetrated his clothes and hands while he was in the laboratory. His friend wrinkled her nose and said, "Why don't you become a doctor?"

From such a source, this was a weighty suggestion. It became irresistible when the young man discovered that the woman's father shared her wish, and would even pay the costs of medical school. One suspects a conspiracy. Perhaps the potential father-in-law even hatched the plot. In any event the deal was carried out and it pleased all parties.

Young people seeking a professional education commonly debate the merits of a life in medicine versus a life at law. Fathers who are doctors or lawyers may offer some strong opinions on this choice. In the 1880s a father favoring law advised his son: "If you will be practicing law you will be sitting in a comfortable office and your client will come to you; but if you practice medicine you will have to go to them — at all hours of the day and night, and in all kinds of weather, on all kinds of roads, and to all kinds of people. Further, if you practice law you will have an intelligent man to be your judge, but if you practice medicine you will be judged by every damned fool in the country."

This debate was updated in 1968. Surgeon William Nolan wrote that his career choice was heavily influenced by his father who was a lawyer. "If you're smart," his father advised, "when you grow up you'll be a doctor. Those bastards have it made."

What would Oliver Wendell Holmes have thought of that? Holmes, our "Autocrat of the Breakfast Table" (1809-1894), spent a year in the Harvard Law School and then switched to medicine. He was subsequently the professor of anatomy at Harvard and then dean of the medical school. Aside from being disquieted by the infelicity of the language, Holmes would be astonished by the judgment. Holmes was adamant that neither of his sons follow him into medicine. "I expect both my boys to become lawyers," he said. And Oliver Wendell Holmes Jr. became a distinguished justice of the United States Supreme Court.

One might be tempted to conclude that in the last century medicine has so distinguished itself by new discoveries that it has risen from being a disdained profession to equal or surpass law as a career choice by the young. But we tend to find obvious reasons in retrospect for decisions and pursuits that were subtle and complex in origin — perhaps even made without reason. Dr. Carl Wiggers was chairman of the admissions committee of Western Reserve University Medical School in the 1940s. He routinely asked applicants, "Why do you want to be a physician?" The answers were never quite satisfying, he said. And of himself he added, "I never chose medicine as a profession; I drifted into it."

Perhaps the most encompassing, widely applicable answer to the question is the one given by the physician who said, "Why I ever wanted to be a doctor is a mystery to me."

3.

The Fabric of Man

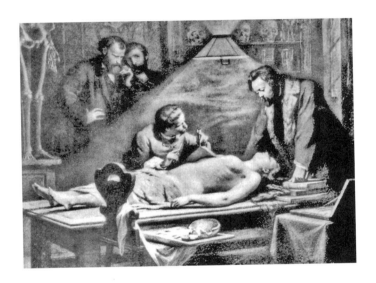

When medical schools were established in America — the first was in Philadelphia in 1765 — a difficulty arose immediately: How were bodies going to be obtained for anatomical studies? There were no laws to permit an orderly acquisition of cadavers for such studies. Grave robbing came to the Colonies. Anatomy professors took to grave robbing to provide material for their classes and "resurrectionists" appeared: individuals who provided bodies to the schools for a fee. When these practices were exposed, the public reaction was violent.

The resurrectionists usually obtained their bodies from the graveyards, but a few are known to have resorted to murder. Intermediate methods were often quite ingenious. A Boston surgeon told about a man who suddenly fell dead on a busy street. A resurrectionist who was passing saw opportunity and intervened swiftly. He said that the fallen man was his brother and he took charge of the body. He transported the corpse to a nearby dissection theatre and sold it promptly for a good price.

Wags wrote verses about the resurrectionists. This one, the lament of a recently buried corpse circulated widely:

The body-snatchers they have come
And made a snatch at me
It's very hard them kind of men
Won't let a body be!
Don't go to weep upon my grave
And think that there I be
They haven't left an atom there
Of my anatomy.

Some towns employed grave watchers, armed men who guarded new graves for some ten nights, after which the body would be unfit for anatomical study. When a grave was reported to have been disturbed, families who had nearby cemetery plots were known to dig up the caskets of their relatives to be sure that they were still there. Some families buried members in their gardens rather than risk a cemetery, and a few placed the grave just beneath a window of the house where they were likely to be alerted if the grave was disturbed.

In winter, bodies were sometimes stored in churches because the ground was frozen. They would be buried in the spring. But the resurrectionists invaded the churches. Some churches established iron-barred safe rooms where bodies could be kept until they were unsuitable for dissection.

Some of the early medical schools did not teach anatomy. The need was obvious, but the schools were unable to fulfill it. Conscientious graduates sought ways to supplement their education. When Dr. James Douglas opened his practice in Utica, New York, in 1823, he knew very little about anatomy. He obtained a cadaver and dissected for knowledge in a small room above his office. His activity became known and he was threatened with jail. A forthright plea to the local judge on the absolute necessity of anatomical education resolved the matter. But the judge warned against any repetition of such behavior.

About a year later, Dr. Douglas raided a grave for another body. His endeavor took a bad turn when a patient, looking for the doctor when he was out, wandered into the dissecting room and recognized the body under study there. The patient promised secrecy, but the doctor was wary. He reburied the body the same night and left town early in the morning.

In 1838 an Indiana doctor encountered similar difficulties in his quest for anatomical knowledge. He was brought into court and charged with bringing about "a premature resurrection of two Indians." He wanted the skeletons in order to study the bones.

In the medical schools that did teach anatomy, the professors involved themselves in some exciting affairs when they undertook to provide the necessary teaching material. Dr. Joseph Nash McDowell was the professor of anatomy at Cincinnati College, a medical school opened in 1835. He was a busy resurrectionist and he seemed to enjoy the dangers it involved, but he surely had second thoughts on one occasion. McDowell had exhumed the body of a young female and transported it to the college laboratory.

The theft was discovered almost immediately, and McDowell was followed by outraged family members and mob of supportive friends.

This angry group, armed with rifles and carrying a rope for a hanging, surrounded the college anatomy building and forced an entry. McDowell was in the building; he was cornered. He quickly secured the corpse from its table and hoisted it into the attic. Then he mounted the empty table, drew the sheet — one covered each cadaver— up over his head and tried to breathe as shallowly as possible.

McDowell's pursuers rushed into the dissection room and out of it again looking for him. One angry man paused at the table where the professor was hiding , and remarked, "Here's one who died with his boots on," but he was disinclined to raise the sheet — McDowell escaped.

Some public raids on the medical schools were more successful. In 1830 a fiery group of three hundred men, aroused by a grave-robbing, entered a medical school at Castleton, Vermont, recovered the body they sought and returned it to its grave. Another such affair was concluded in a droll vein. A disinterred body was recovered from a medical school near Pittsfield, Massachusetts, in 1840. Forty persons had attended the first funeral; six hundred attended the reburial.

In one instance a tombstone was even erected to commemorate a grave-robbing event. In Hoosick Falls, New York, in 1846, the resurrected corpse of a girl, which had been partially dissected, was rescued and reburied. Her tombstone was then inscribed:

> *Her body dissected by fiendish men*
> *Her bones anatomized*
> *Her soul we trust has risen to God*
> *Where few physicians rise.*

As additional medical schools were established, public apprehension mounted. Charters for the establishment of new schools were opposed by citizen groups; body-snatching would surely follow. To allay concern, colleges in small communities assured the citizens that the bodies used for their anatomical studies would be obtained from large cities, at great distances — never locally. The city colleges averred that their anatomical material would come from the remote countryside — never from the city.

Most cadavers came from the vicinity of the school. Potters' fields were favored by the resurrectionists; persons buried there usually had no known relatives or interested friends. When more than one medical school was within snatching distance of such a ground, the schools might make a gentleman's agreement to attend new graves alternately. A few bodies were shipped about, from New York City to New England, for instance, pickled in barrels of brine labeled beef, pork or pickles or in barrels of whisky.

Citizens became suspicious of hospitals, especially public hospitals. In the late 1800s the great Philadelphia public hospital familiarly known as Blockly (4,000 beds) had an unwarranted reputation among African Americans for murdering patients in order to provide bodies for dissection. Doctors who wanted autopsies in order to learn from special patients were lumped with the resurrectionists and dissectors. Alexsis St. Martin was such a patient. He had suffered a gunshot wound of the abdomen that did not heal completely; his stomach could be observed through the unhealed area.

Doctors had their first opportunity to study gastric functions directly. Dr. William Osier was known to be very interested in obtaining an autopsy when St. Martin died, to put a cap on these studies. But when St. Martin died the local physician sent a telegram to Dr. Osier, "Don't come for autopsy," he said, "Will be killed." Relatives guarded the grave for days.

Medical students often assisted their professors at graverobbing. It was well known that they did. So they were often referred to as "grave rats." When Ambrose Bierce published *The Devil's Dictionary* (1911), he defined 'grave' as "A place in which the dead are laid to await the coming of the medical student."

Dr. George Crile, a founder of the prestigious Cleveland Clinic, related how as a student he accompanied the professor of anatomy of the Wooster Medical School in Cleveland on nighttime expeditions to pauper graves. Crile wrote that it was psychologically the most difficult thing he had ever done. Excavating the grave was easy enough, but handling the body was most unpleasant. He described driving through Cleveland on a moonless night with a properly dressed "stiff" propped upright in a carriage between himself and the professor of anatomy.

When bodies were in short supply, the students complained; they were paying dear fees for instruction. At Harvard in 1870 an instructor with a wry sense of humor responded to the complaints of his students: "I assure you gentlemen," he said, "I have left no stone unturned to unearth a subject."

In Washington a few years later, a cadaver shortage stimulated student enterprise. Five medical students formed the Hippocratic Exhumation Corporation, an organization to provide a steady supply of cadavers and, simultaneously, funds for student education — their own.

The students searched the newspapers for death notices. Then they sent out an "advance man" who paid a visit of condolence to the home of the bereaved, inquired into the cause of death, the day of burial and the cemetery. One of the group attended the funeral and recorded the grave site in relation to nearby landmarks. The organization functioned effectively for three years.

Grave-robbing set the stage for other curious incidents. A tale from Cincinnati tells of a student who encountered his father's corpse on his dissecting table. In Baltimore a student found his sister's corpse in the anatomy hall. But recognition might be difficult. Another incident involved the arrival of a sheriff at an anatomy laboratory; he was accompanied by a young man and they came to reclaim the body of the young man's father — it had been exhumed. The proper body was viewed, but to the great relief of the anatomists, the young man failed to recognize it. He said it was not his father. The post-mortem changes confused and misled him.

The early professors of anatomy were a devoted group of men. Dr. John Collins Warren, who became professor of anatomy at the Harvard Medical School in 1815, devoted himself to it literally. In his will he provided that his skeleton be articulated and hung in the school's medical museum as a teaching tool.

It is still in the Harvard museum. Every medical school anatomy laboratory had a caretaker, usually a stoical, cynical type, often devoted to spirits, always full of stories and much respected by the medical students. In the mid-nineteenth century the medical school at Louisville, Kentucky, was considered the greatest in the West. The caretaker at the Louisville school also supplied the bodies for the anatomy studies. How he got them, no one knew.

His name was Pete. The students dubbed him "St. Peter," and jovially maintained that he was the rock upon which the anatomical church was founded and the one to whom the keys of the cemetery had been given.

At the Missouri Medical College in St. Louis during the 1890s, the caretaker of the anatomy hall was as highly regarded as any member of the faculty. "He was the only person connected with the college who knew us all by name," a doctor recalled. He cared for the building, the cadavers, the skeletons and the pathological specimens. If a lecturer was late the caretaker might address the class. He was a good speaker and even handed out the diplomas in some years with appropriate remarks to each student.

The University of Pennsylvania once had a similar paragon. Dr. Howard Rush told how when he graduated in 1925 he hoped to leave Philadelphia immediately. But commencement was held three weeks after graduation and the university refused to award a degree to any student who was not present to accept it. The janitor of the animal house kept a cap and gown for just such dilemmas. For five dollars he would don the cap and gown, receive the degree and mail the diploma. He had received more medical degrees than anyone in the country. This solution worked well for Dr. Rusk, but at a class reunion some years later, a classmate joshed Dr. Rush about how fumbling drunk he had been at commencement. The janitor seems to have fortified himself a bit for his performance.

In the course of the nineteenth century, successive states passed Anatomy Acts that made legal provisions for the acquisition of certain unclaimed bodies by the medical schools. The resurrectionists were no longer called upon.

Anatomy is the medical student's most difficult subject because of the mass of detail that is involved and the circumstances in which it must be mastered. The first requirement is adaptation to the odor of the dissecting hall. A student described it at the Louisville medical school in 1900: "I had grown up on a farm — putrid flesh and bad odors were not new to me, but the dissecting room outstripped all the unpleasant experiences of my life and taught me to smoke in self-defense."

In the early schools dissection was done only during the cool seasons of the year; tissue putrefaction made it otherwise impossible. Various methods of cadaver preservation were tried before preservation in a solution of formaldehyde became the prevailing one. Cadavers could be preserved in formaldehyde and dissected at any time. But at dissection, formaldehyde fumes wafted upward from the cadavers causing the student's eyes to water and noses to smart. The disagreeable combined odor of flash and formaldehyde penetrated the dissectors' clothing and skin and remained there to be augmented on the following day. No amount of washing would remove it. An anatomy student came to smell exactly like his cadaver. At meals the odor of one's hands overwhelmed the taste of the food. On streetcars people moved to another seat. Pet cats and dogs turned away. Jesters named the scent "Eau de Cadavre." Some students selected a single set of clothes to wear in the anatomy hall and burned the clothes at the end of the course.

Slowed by the increasing intensity of the odor and fumes, students approached their cadavers cautiously. The first assignment was usually a dissection of the muscles of the back. But the cadaver might be lying face up on the table. Dissection would be delayed while the students pondered the ways to turn the cadaver over; until they finally decided that the only way to do it was to wrap their arms around it, hold it close and turn it.

A few other preliminaries might be required before dissection began. A contemporary young lady told of some in a letter she wrote home describing her first week in medical school. She addressed her mother, but when she told about her anatomy class she changed the addressee: "Now you better turn this over to Daddy or you'll get sick.... Daddy, my cadaver is a six foot, forty-seven year old male.... we had to scrape off all the grease coating with a scalpel, shave all the body hair and wash the body with soap and water.... nearly vomited.... God does he stink!"

The impact of the anatomy laboratory can be profound and long-lasting. Dr. Joseph Leidy told of his introduction to anatomy as a student in 1840: "I was so disgusted with the dissection room that after spending the first half-day there, I went away and could not be induced to return for nearly six weeks, and I did not get entirely over the melancholy produced for a year."

But he seems to have been helpless in the hands of destiny. In 1853 he became professor of anatomy at the University of Pennsylvania and his research and teaching in the field made him one of the luminaries of American medical history.

Usually the adjustment to the dissecting room is quick and gratifying. George Middleton described his engagement at a Baltimore medical college in 1892: "The first contact with the dissecting room was a revolting experience. To see human bodies handled as we handle logs of wood, carved up like butcher's meat and pickled in vats for future use seemed certainly an antithesis of the Scripture... Strange to say, however, a few days later I was working in the dissecting room with all the fervor of an enthusiastic student."

Professors sought to set an elevated and solemn tone in their anatomy laboratories. One at the University of Louisville opened the session with a skeleton hanging at his side as he recited a verse titled "Ode to the Skeleton." It is an anonymous verse, Shakespearean in tenor. He began with the skull:

Behold this ruin! It is a skull
Once of ethereal spirit full
This narrow cell was life's retreat
This space was thought's mysterious seat
Within this hollow cavern hung
The ready, swift and tuneful tongue

Students were likely to treat anatomy less solemnly. They preferred a verse in which anatomic study is construed as a love affair between the student and his cadaver. She is "Brown Cadavera" (cadavers tend to become brown and leathery) the medical student's inamorata:

I have loved
Brown Cadavera did my soul ensnare
And in a secret hour approached her grave
Resolved her precious corpse from worms to save
With active haste remov'd the incumbent clay
Seized the rich prize and bore my love away
Her naked charms now lay before my sight
I gaz'd with rapture and supreme delight
Nor could forbear, in ecstasy to cry
Beneath that shrivili'd skin what treasures lie!
Then feasted to the full my amorous soul
And skinned and cut and slashed without control
My true love's bones I boiled — from fat and lean
And ev'ry bone did to its place restore
Now what remains of Cadavera mine
Hangs securely in a case of pine.

There was so much to be learned about bones and the attachments of muscles to bones that the medical schools made it a practice to supply each student with a box of more than a hundred skeletal bones for study. It required a box about two-and-a-half feet long and a foot high to contain the collection. The students could then take the bones to their rooms for study. The students misplaced the boxes at times: forgot them on streetcars, in lavatories and eateries, causing great excitement when a box was discovered and a horrible crime suspected. The police in our large cities became quite familiar with the medical students' boxes of bones.

The boxes of bones caused other odd incidents. Esther Lovejoy, the first woman to graduate from the medical school of the University of Oregon, worked in a department store part-time to support herself in school. She worked at the women's underwear counter. She studied her anatomy book in the intervals between customers and referred to a few bones which she kept hidden in the underwear. The floorwalker noticed the bones amid the underwear and Esther Lovejoy was fired.

Students coveted skeletons for private study and obtained them in various surreptitious ways. In Boston a student aspiring to surgery obtained a skeleton and hung it in his boarding house closet. A chambermaid opened the closet door and fell to the floor in hysterics when she confronted the skeleton.

Dissection by the students was often preceded by one or more demonstration dissections conducted by the professor. Dr. Thomas Dwight, a professor of anatomy at Harvard, liked to tease his students when he dissected in front of a new class. He pretended to cut his finger and after expressing both alarm and dismay he would turn to the class and say, "When you cut yourself you always want suck it." Then he brought a clean, protected finger to his mouth and proceeded to do so. Usually at least one student keeled over; the rest were left startled and confused, pondering the veracity of the advice for the rest of the session.

In the 1870s the dissection hall at the University of Virginia had a great pit at one end, some forty feet deep, in which anatomical fragments and ultimately the dissected bodies were disposed of. On the wall over the pit an artist with a great sense of humor had depicted the confusion that would arise on Judgment Day as a result of the studies carried on in this hall. He painted a large mural showing a profusion of anatomical parts ascending from the pit and reassembling with great disorder. Incomplete bodies hunted for the various missing parts they needed. A female figure missing a large leg bone was shown being assisted by a male with an armful of similar bones; he seemed hopeful that one of them might fit her. Another pair searched through an assortment of bones for appropriate parts that they needed. It appeared that the resurrection was causing infinite chaos; the theme was worthy of Michelangelo.

A knowledge of anatomy alters a student's world forever. Anatomical features are seen in places where they were never noticed before, in foods for instance. Some things that were formerly consumed with gusto might suddenly become unapproachable.

One first year medical student, burdened by the heavy study schedule and deprived for weeks of any social engagements, was delighted to be invited out for weekend dinner at a chop house — she needed diversion. To her dismay she found herself staring at a "beautiful thick mutton chop, unable to eat it because there, nestled together, I see the cross-section of an artery, vein and nerve exactly as they are seen in the anatomy lab. My God! I am looking at the sacro-spinal muscle of a sheep."

And Dr. James Newton described how one's perception of a pretty girlfriend might change.

Just back of the light of her eyes
Just under the pink other hands

Whose velvet the lily out-vies
A skeleton stands.

Beneath the gold crown other tress
And the clustering gems she wears
And under the silks that caress
A skeleton stares.
Her laughter is that of a lover
Her lips are as lush as the South
And I shudder to think they but cover
A skeleton's mouth.

Most such revulsions subside quickly. In a few weeks a woman might park a bag of brownies beside her cadaver and share them with her cadaver-mates. The students might trade favorite recipes as they worked.

The young men devised humorous names for their cadavers and passed off-color jokes from table to table.

When one has accommodated to the milieu of anatomical studies, the complexity and magnitude of the subject causes new anguish: How does one master this multitude of minutiae? The assimilation of anatomy is a wellspring of mnemonics.

Mnemonics are senseless constructions, words, or phrases, the first letters of which — or in the case of phrases the first letter of each word — call to mind some related bits of information. "BITEM" is a useful and amusing anatomical mnemonic. It calls up the names of the muscles of mastication, the chewing and biting muscles. They are small muscles, seldom necessary to think about, but on occasion very important, an element of anatomical knowledge that must be available on demand. BITEM calls them to mind and in the anatomical order in which they are arranged in the body: buccinator, internal pterygoid, temporal, external pterygoid, and masseter muscles.

Many mnemonics are smutty, devised by students to

facilitate recall at the time of examinations; vulgarities stick in the memory. There is "Never Lower Tillie's Pants, Mother May Come Home." It recalls the names of the bones of the wrist — a group of quite similar, tiny structures: navicular, lunate, triangular, etc. "Not Tonight, Please," recalls the anatomical structures passing through a pelvic opening, and there is "Some Inherit Money, Others Inherit Insanity," which clues a student to the names of the branches of an important artery.

In the days before modem, hospital-based, surgical training programs, young medical graduates who hoped to be surgeons continued their anatomical studies at night in the medical school laboratories or in the city morgues, wherever they could induce a caretaker to cooperate.

Dr. John Wyeth aspired to surgery; he dissected in the morgue of Bellevue Hospital during the nighttimes of 1873. He was often very tired, having worked a full day before turning to his anatomical studies. On one occasion he dissected the structures of the axilla (the armpit). He was seated beside the cadaver and he paused to rest his head for a moment on his own outstretched arm, which rested on his subject's chest. He dozed, and as he did, the weight of his head and his arm compressed the cadaver's chest and slowly expressed the air from its lungs. As Wyeth awakened he drew his arm off the cadaver's chest and as the ribs rose, the chest expanded and drew air into the lungs causing a wheezing, gurgling sound as the air passed through the throat. Half asleep, Wyeth was terrified: he was gripped by a fear that his subject was alive! Then his head cleared and the circumstances were evident.

Philadelphia surgeon William Keen related a similar experience in a morgue. On one occasion he made a scalp incision in a first step to exposing the brain and his knife passed through the ends of muscles attached to the jaws. The muscle irritation caused the corpse to open and close its jaw several times in quick succession and each closure was associated with a sharp clack of the teeth. A frightened morgue attendant exclaimed, "Good God! Isn't he dead?" Dr. Keen said that he shuddered when he recalled the event, even after fifty years.

Professors of anatomy exert themselves to allay apprehension among the students when a new group arrives to begin dissection studies. They devise some amusing ways of doing so. One of our major medical schools recently scheduled a day before the opening of regular class work on which new students could come to the anatomy laboratory and "meet" their cadavers. The students were given a card with a table number and entry to the lab where some thirty covered corpses rested on tables. No teacher was present. The "meeting" consisted of finding the proper table and raising the cover from the grim visage of the designated corpse. Whoever devised that exercise exhibited, unwittingly to be sure, a marvelous sense of humor.

4.
Babies

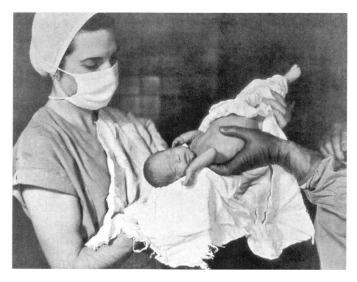

Just arrived

Prior to the Revolutionary War, American babies were delivered by midwives. Except among the affluent in the large cities, midwives fulfilled this role until the time of the Civil War and in some areas they were busy through the first half of the twentieth century. But there were many instances where women who were not midwives fulfilled this role for members of their own family or for friends. A mother might be the midwife to her daughter, her daughter-in-law, her granddaughter and her sister.

Cleveland's Dr. George Crile told how an elderly, black midwife gave him his first lesson in obstetrics in 1885. Crile was a young teacher in an Ohio village; he thought he might like to be a doctor. A friendly physician encouraged him; he invited Crile to accompany and assist him when he made his rounds.

One of the doctor's patients was about to have a baby; she was the village Magdalene, and the doctor invited Crile to assist at the birth. George Crile had never witnessed a birth; he looked forward to it with great anticipation and studied a book on obstetrics assiduously to prepare himself for the event.

When labor began, Crile was delegated to watch the expectant mother while his physician-tutor went about his calls. A mother's distress in labor can be an alarming affair for a neophyte, and after enduring it for several hours, Crile was immensely relieved when a fragile, elderly midwife joined the vigil.

The doctor had involved her as an assistant when his own availability became uncertain. Two additional hours passed and the crisis seemed near, but Crile could think of nothing useful to do. The old midwife calmed his rising anxiety: "Well, Doc," she said, "Don't you think we'd better quill her?"

Crile had no idea what she meant, but she obviously knew something that he did not, and it seemed best to signal approval. The midwife brought forth a quill (the barrel of a bird's feather) and a packet of snuff from the little bag that she carried. She filled the quill with snuff, put one end in the laboring mother's nose and her own mouth to the other end; then she blew sharply into the quill. The mother responded immediately with a tremendous sneeze and Crile wrote that "to my astonishment the baby arrived precipitately,"

The technique was common among midwives. Babies precipitated into the world in this manner were often referred to as "quilled babies" for years afterward. The midwives also spoke of "snuffing out," the same procedure, or of "sneezing her.".". Many of the midwives chewed snuff, so it was readily available.

The arrival of a baby was a social event among the early settlers. Where the proximity of neighbors permitted it, the ladies gathered to assume the household chores, socialize, and in the event that a midwife or a doctor was not available, to assist at the birth. A rural doctor of the early period described a delivery he attended: "I found my patient reclining in a small room containing a fireplace, two beds and five neighborhood women.... who had with them three small babies and two dogs."

The gatherings for a baby's arrival were referred to as "frolics." Not to be invited to an entertainment of this kind was an offense not easily forgiven. One account relates that "no sooner was the cry of the newborn baby heard than the rattling of dishes in the adjoining room became evident and soon we were all invited in.... And such a dinner!"

Childbirth is a mysterious affair in the minds of children and the midwives perpetuated the mystery. A well-known one in Pennsylvania always arrived with her hands under her apron if there were young children in the home, as though she was carrying something. She went directly to the room of the expecting mother. Later, the children would be told that she "brought" the new baby.

At the time of the Revolutionary War, premarital conceptions ran as high as 35 percent in some areas of the country. Many of these situations were rescued by very late marriages. One young man called and demanded to see his girl friend who was in labor. He was told it was impossible — the baby might be born any minute. He didn't care; he was going to marry her; it was all arranged and it could be done only a half mile away. She was bundled up, transported, married, and brought back just in time to deliver the baby.

In another instance a pregnant teenager was prevented from marrying by local laws though the boy involved was quite willing to marry her. When she was finally old enough to marry, they did marry. At that time the baby was two years old.

For a time Massachusetts had an amusing law designed to deal with out of wedlock conceptions. The law required that the midwife exhort the unwed mother to name the father of the child during labor.

The name was to be demanded at the peak of the labor pains when it was thought that the mother's distress would make her most likely to speak the truth. The practice was soon abandoned.

In 1762 Dr. William Shippen, a Philadelphian who had studied medicine abroad, urged American physicians to attend expectant mothers and to assist at childbirth. A few doctors had already done so, but the idea was generally ridiculed — man midwives? Some thought that the idea was comical, but most thought that it was wicked: an invasion that would destroy the modesty of American womanhood.

But the change came about because the lives of mothers and babies lost in the birth process could sometimes be saved if a doctor was present. But a hundred years passed before the practice was generally accepted.

When the first medical schools were established, the students were given lectures on childbirth, but the schools could not provide their students with experience. Conscientious students would sometimes persuade a woman who was seen in the dispensary to let the professor deliver her before the class. Class members pitched in fifty cents each to finance the demonstration; half of the money went to the obliging woman and half to a hospital for her brief stay.

Some students would persuade a woman who was having her second or third child to let them deliver her at home; she knew more about it than they did and she usually told them how to do it. Dr. Joseph DeLee, Chicago's first great obstetrician, graduated from the Chicago Medical College in 1891 and began to practice obstetrics having seen — through opera glasses — two women deliver their babies in the amphitheater of the college.

To provide their students with experience, the medical schools began to send the students out to assist at home deliveries. The schools provided a service to the community and the students acquired experience. The schools' doctors selected women who had already had at least one baby and were thought to pose little risk of complications. The students were instructed to be alert for difficulties and to call for help if things did not go smoothly.

Beginning in the mid-1800s, medical students became thoroughly acquainted with the streets and courts of the slums in all of our large cities as they delivered the babies in those sections. Prowling about in the tenement districts at night was dangerous. It was difficult to find addresses and obvious perplexity attracted muggers. In Boston, a doctor who dispatched Harvard students on home deliveries in 1908 alarmed them facetiously by asking, "Whom shall I notify in case of an accident?"

But generally the students were recognized by the bags they carried and given a safe passage. In one incident a student was assaulted and his watch taken. On the following morning two men appeared in the hospital dining room and proffered the watch. "We didn't know you were from the hospital," they said.

Appearances were important for the student obstetricians. At the University of Pennsylvania, the student making home obstetrical calls was obliged to wear the "Obstetrical Hat," All doctors wore high hats in those days, and for fear that the student might not receive the proper respect and cooperation, an appropriate high hat was provided as part of the student's equipment.

When the proper apartment was located, it was common to find several female relatives and often a few neighbors as well, flying about the room in various stages of agitation over the anticipated event. The first rule of a set of admonitions given to the students dealt with this gathering of females:

"The first thing to do is to determine which of the assembled ladies is going to have the baby."

The second rule was a bit of black humor indulged in by the interns who had survived the anxieties of home deliveries and were now supervising the students: "If the blood pools on the mattress, everything is alright; if it drips on the floor you may be in trouble; if it runs downstairs, call me."

This levity did not imply any lack of concern for the mother, indeed it implied just the opposite: it was meant to reassure the student who was as likely as any layman to be unsettled by the sight of blood.

The early Harvard students attending home deliveries were given what came to be called the "Panic Slip." It was a slip on which they could write the nature of the problem if they required help. They were to send the husband back to the hospital with the slip. One student sent his panic slip back with the imprint of a bloody hand on it and the single word "Hemorrhage." Another student wrote, "Something is bulging, I know not what." One sent a husband back with instructions on the slip for the intern to hold him; he was annoying and troublesome, the student wrote.

Though the students and interns were generally well treated, inevitably there were some alarming incidents. In New York when an Italian mother fainted away in the course of a long labor her husband thought she was dead. He drew a knife to kill the doctor, but was restrained by relatives — all of this behind an intern's back. Then the mother aroused and sobbed that she wanted her "bambino," and the father collapsed. The intern wrote that if an aria, sung in Italian, could have been added to the scene it would have equalled any staged at the Metropolitan Opera.

Life was harsh in the tenement rooms. One student had his pocket picked while he was assisting at a delivery. He put his coat over a chair and the patient's husband went through it while the baby was being born. The student found a policeman, pursued the man to a nearby saloon and recovered his wallet. In Boston, a female student took off her underwear because there was nothing else available in which to wrap the baby. The students sought to hang their coats inside the nurses' cloaks (if there was a nurse), otherwise fleas invaded the coats. One laboring patient was thought to be delirious. She called out repeatedly: "Eyes!" But a look upward revealed three sets of eyes looking down between the ceiling boards.

Beneficent institutions made touching efforts to cushion a baby's entry into this trying world. The obstetrical bag of one New York hospital (carried by the students) included a half-pint of whisky to be dispensed as thought fit — usually to the father — and two-and-a-half dollars for coal or any other necessity that the family might lack for the care of the baby. The students marveled that "in a filthy room, a pit of drunken noise, obscenity and wife-beating, the magical was accomplished: a perfect baby was born."

Students learned that the timing of an infant's arrival could be difficult to predict. At the University of Texas in the early 1900s, students were sent out on home deliveries in pairs. One such team arrived at the bedside of a young lady having her first baby and things were progressing very slowly. It seemed likely that several hours would pass before the students could play any role. They left the bedside to get a cup of coffee a few doors down the street. The baby arrived while they were away.

Or they might arrive too late. One student on a home delivery arrived to find the mother asleep, the baby beside her still attached to the umbilical cord and its one-year-old sister trying to induce it to play.

Even if a student's arrival and presence were appropriately timed, a neophyte might still never get things quite under control. A student engaged in his first home delivery in Philadelphia in 1869 "arrived just in time —1 will not say to deliver — but rather to be present." He washed his hands, scrubbed his nails thoroughly and then made what he thought would be a preliminary examination of his patient. But "before I could go over in my mind what to do at the proper time and manner, I found a slippery baby in the bed."

A neighbor woman was present, and while the student was "endeavoring now to recall the precise instruction" he had received about tying off the umbilical cord, the neighbor noticed what he was failing to note and exclaimed, "'My, My, there's another!' And to my surprise and confusion the neighbor was right"

The problem of timing the doctor to the baby has resisted solution, but most mothers seem to be no worse off because of it.

At the turn of the last century, a doctor in Oklahoma told of arriving too late to be of any assistance and no other assistance had been available. But the mother had reached into her nearby sewing basket and found an appropriate thread with which to tie the umbilical cord and used her sewing scissors to cut it.

And it was an experienced doctor, Dr. David Kellogg of Plattsburgh, New York, not a student, who perhaps set the record for arriving too late: "I had a peculiar experience yesterday and last night. A man came for me about 7:30 in the morning and wanted me to go to his home in a hurry. I hurried and was there in about 25 minutes, but a baby was born before I got there.

"About half past 10 p.m. another man came and wanted me to go to his home in a hurry. I dressed quickly and was at his home in about 20 minutes, but a boy was born before I got there.

"About 1 this a.m. a man came to the house and thought he might want me to go his house soon. I advised him to go back and if he needed me I would go quickly. He returned soon and I was at his home before two o'clock. But before I reached his home, two boys were born."

Occasionally a recent immigrant made a home delivery simple and quick. On one tenement obstetrical call in New York in the early 1900s, the woman who answered the door was a Bohemian cigarette maker who did not speak English. When the nature of the visit was explained, she nodded and motioned the doctor to a comfortable chair. Then she resumed rolling cigarettes at her work chair, which had one flat arm bearing a small pile of tobacco, a pack of papers and a small knife. She rolled cigarettes, clearly in considerable pain at times, but doggedly determined to persist in her task as long as possible. She worked on for the best part of an hour. Then she rose from her chair, motioned the doctor toward the bed as she moved to it, reclined on the bed and delivered the baby immediately.

But a lack of communication might create problems. In Chicago in 1929 a student made a home-delivery call to the apartment of an Italian family. He found an 18-year-old in labor. The girl had been born in Chicago and spoke English, but a grandmother who did not speak English was obviously in charge.

Students were taught to shun vaginal examinations for fear of causing infection; the state and progress of a delivery can be gauged very well by means of a rectal examination. The Chicago student conducted a rectal examination and determined that delivery was not imminent. After a suitable period he examined the laboring girl again. After each of these examinations there was a sharp verbal exchange between the girl and an obviously agitated grandmother. After another waiting period the student approached the girl for a third time and the grandmother exploded in a torrent of words that seemed to have no end. The expectant mother responded by holding up her hand. "Stop," she said, "You're not a doctor. My grandmother said you don't even know where babies come from."

Home deliveries exposed the students to marvelous bits of wisdom buried in folklore: practices not to be found in any medical textbook. Another Chicago student was called to an Italian section of the city in the 1930s to see a young lady who was about to have her first child and whose relatives were gathered to celebrate the event. He was introduced to Maria and he determined that she was harboring a large baby above some very small hip bones: a small pelvis. She was in labor, but it seemed doubtful that she could deliver the baby; a Cesarean operation might well be necessary.

The girl's mother had delivered nine babies with scarcely a groan, and her grandmother had delivered ten. Adding to this family was a routine affair, and dallying over the matter was not good form. Maria dallied in a shameful way. The relatives bore it well, but after about fifteen hours of eating spaghetti and drinking Chianti they grew impatient for the climax of the celebration.

The student doctor thought that the birth process had stalled: the girl had been given a lengthy trial; a Cesarean operation was indicated.

When he expressed his opinion there was an uproar among the relatives; grandmother threatened violence if he interfered with nature's course in any way. The difficulty was explained to the one relative who understood English and conveyed to the belligerent grandmother. As soon as the grandmother understood the reason for the delay, she knew what to do and she took charge.

Pushing the medical student aside, the grandmother marshaled the forces present to hoist the mother to a standing position on a table. This done, she motioned everyone to stand back. "One, two, three, jump!" she commanded and the pregnant girl floated into space before the eyes of the horrified medical student and shook the building when she landed on the floor. Despite her screams, the girl was gathered up and set on the table again, "One, two, three, jump!" The grandmother umpired and the medical student lost track of the innings. But ultimately a moment came when the grandmother pointed at the prostrate mother on the floor and to an emerging baby, "See," she said. "Doctors know nothing."

The method has very limited application and one would

not expect to ever hear of it again. But in 1984 an American doctor encountered it in China. He cared for a mother through a prolonged labor, tried every maneuver he knew to deliver the baby including an attempt at delivery with forceps — everything failed.

The doctor again commanded a Cesarean operation but the family refused. They resorted to "Chunging." Two women each seized one arm of the expectant mother, lifted her up and jounced her down violently and repeatedly, as if to shake the baby out. And they did. Much to the doctor's surprise a healthy baby emerged, none the worse for the violence that attended its arrival.

Students on home deliveries encountered other practices for which their lectures had not prepared them. The students showed marvelous adaptability, and one young woman left an entertaining image of doing so. She encountered a mother-to-be who labored in a standing position; her pains seemed easier to endure when she was standing and she wanted to continue that way. The student was a paragon of accommodative assistance: "Trying to be where I could best take care of the baby as it came out and down between her legs, I lay on the floor under her facing upward between her legs." A step by step account of what followed is lacking — a lamentable misfortune for the history of humor in medicine.

The image of this incident must be paired with another that was created in San Diego when a Mexican woman crossed the border to have her baby in an American hospital and a medical student, assigned to his first delivery, was her attendant. The student was astonished and alarmed when in the midst of labor his patient suddenly sat up and then stood on her bed in a semi-squatting position. He was utterly unprepared to assist a mother in this remarkable position. He dashed off for a nurse and returned with one in less than a minute; he found the perfect simile to describe what they saw when they entered the room: "We saw Mrs. Cortez from behind, all 4 feet 8 inches of her compact body working to extrude her son, whose head now faced us from below her hips. The pair of them looked like a long lost Mayan deity with two heads, at once able to see forward and backward, right side up and upside down."

Newborns are hardy little beings and it is well that they are because they are subjected to a long list of incredible accidental insults. If labor seemed to stall, a resourceful student might administer an enema. The impulses that arise to expel the enema stimulate the resumption of labor and the delivery of the baby. A student in Chicago elected to try this method when labor ceased during a home delivery in the 1930s. But when an enema is given, a mother may perceive only one great impulse to evacuate and so it was with this student's subject. When the mother expelled the enema into the tenement slop jar the baby tumbled into the same receptacle. A swift rescue was accomplished and after "much washing and reassurance" the baby and mother were well and content.

Dr. William Osier, the sage of Johns Hopkins, gathered the facts about a baby whose entry into the world was one of the most unpromising on record. In this instance a mother accommodated an urge to use the toilet on a speeding train. The baby who was primarily responsible for this sensation went into the toilet bowl and out the chute onto the bed of the railroad tracks below. The mother realized what had happened, but too late. She immediately had the train stopped and a rescue party hurried back along the tracks looking for the baby. The infant was found, more than a mile back, unharmed except for a few bruises. Dr. Osier wrote an account of this drama for a medical journal, but the editor suspected that the story was a hoax and declined to publish it.

Students can be surprised to learn that a newborn baby is a very slippery creature. In Boston a student successfully assisted a delivery and maneuvered the baby onto his lap as he seated himself at the bedside. The baby immediately slipped off his lap and slid to the floor. The student retrieved it, with some embarrassment, and the same thing happened again. The father exhibited a rapidly rising, ruddy displeasure, but the student was up to the situation. He smiled and said, "Sometimes we have to drop them three times to start them breathing properly."

Is it a boy or a girl? The sex of the newborn brings consternation instead of joy to some parents.

Students learn to deal with this and to judge how much of such a reaction is hyperbole and how much is genuine, and great lessons come from errors of judgment.

When a newborn girl arrived in the apartment of a New York Russian-Jewish couple, the parents were plunged into voluble despair. They wanted a boy. When they were told that a twin was coming they collapsed. The father walked about muttering "Oy vot a trouble!"

Then his wife called him to the bedside; the second child might balance the situation. "Isidore, vot if idt is a Poy?" They both whined and kissed... and kissed and whined. The girl would provide a sister for the boy; boys with sisters were always better boys, they said. But it was another girl.

Isidore was in shock. "He beat his head with his fists... tore out whole handfuls of hair by the roots... and she joined him in the lamentation." The student took it upon himself to humor the parents. "It looked to me like both of them thought death would be sweet compared to the calamity that had befallen them. In a spirit of fun I offered to take the twins back to the hospital and to place them for adoption. Well, I never made a bigger mistake in my life... if looks could kill... both of them forgot all the English they ever knew"

If a delivery became complicated, quick transportation to a hospital was necessary, and many exciting deliveries took place in the ambulances. Student Henry Kessler, famous later for his work in the rehabilitation of men injured in World War II, spent an entire night in 1919 with a woman who was in labor, but did not deliver.

In the early morning he called for an ambulance and accompanied her to the hospital. He tried to encourage the distraught woman: "Be patient, bear up a little, we'll be at the hospital soon." He repeated this encouragement as the ambulance sped along. Suddenly his patient shrieked. Thinking that she was about to deliver, Kessler tried to encourage the process: "Bear down as hard as you can, bear down!" he exhorted. She stopped crying and burst out laughing. "Which is it doctor?" she gasped. "Do you want me to bear up or bear down?"

Among those who did not make it to the hospital delivery room was one young woman who delivered her baby in a hospital elevator. It was a messy, embarrassing, semi-public affair. When it was over, a nurse tried to comfort her: "That's nothing," the nurse said. "Last year a woman gave birth on the front steps of the hospital." And the unlucky mother cried out, "That was me!"

Childbirth moved from the home into the hospital during the first half of the twentieth century.

When it did, nurses became players in the childbirth drama. A nurse might become the principal attendant.

The term "handoff" came into being to describe the circumstances in which the nurse presided. A handoff was a baby delivered by the nurse while the student doctor or intern was getting ready for the delivery.

In a handoff, the nurse handed the baby to the doctor just as he turned toward the mother after finally getting his gown and rubber gloves on.

For the medical student, the impact of assisting the birth process relegated the shock of the anatomy laboratory to the shadows of the mind. The entry of a baby into the world is life's greatest experience: students, nurses and doctors may be as elated by it as the most excited mother. One medical student described her first delivery of a baby as so overwhelming that when the baby gave its first cry she could barely resist an impulse to cry out as well. An intern whose husband was not a doctor described her first experience delivering a baby as so miraculous that "I had to go and tell him all about it and get him up in the middle of the night." And to cap it off a doctor who had delivered 900 babies said that the thrill of the last delivery was equal to the first.

But if the first experience of a student or a nurse involves a difficult or complicated delivery, it is certain to be frightening. Dr. Claude Welch, a professor of surgery at Harvard through the 1960s, told of his and fellow students' reactions to their first-observed deliveries at Harvard in 1930. "During the first observation of such a hair-raising event most students either turned green, had to be assisted from the room by a nurse, or fainted." And of home deliveries he wrote, "These deliveries furnished some of the most memorable and frightening scenes of my life."

Shortly after the Johns Hopkins Hospital opened in 1889, a student nurse attending a birth for the first time in the course of her training assisted at what proved to be a prolonged and perturbing delivery.

When it was over, the nurse disappeared and did not return. She was found sitting in a back stairwell with her head in her hands, tearful and distraught. "Isn't it dreadful, dreadful!" she sobbed. "I'll send back my engagement ring immediately."

If things are difficult during labor, the mood changes promptly when the baby arrives. Some babies arrive with a comical flourish. Obstetricians tell of emerging babies who first thrust one arm through the birth canal, as though exploring the way. One doctor wrote, "I took his hand and ushered him into the world." Or a baby may arrive with its thumb in its mouth, already busy at its favorite pastime. One contemporary baby arrived clutching an intrauterine contraceptive device firmly in its hand as though heralding a triumph of nature over science.

By various methods babies have been observed crying while still in the uterus, yawning, stretching, and even urinating. They have been known to examine the exploring finger of a doctor and even to bite one with well developed front teeth.

Discussions about feeding a baby theorize about a health enhancing "X factor" in breast milk and rhapsodize about the benefits of bonding. Feeding decisions are likely to be more practical. A mother who rejected breast-feeding said it made her feel like a human teething ring. Another who chose breast-feeding said: "Well," referring to her breasts, "If I carry them around I might as well use them."

And the new arrival needs a name. An astonishing number of mothers are not ready with a name for their babies; they solicit the nurses, students and residents in the hospitals. The students and residents are likely to devise whimsical names for their own amusement and they are not beyond foisting one off on an unwary mother. A mother who was a recent immigrant with very little knowledge of English was offered the dulcet euphony of "Anesthesia" as a name for her newborn girl (actually the first baby born under chloroform anesthesia was named Anesthesia). "Euthanasia" might be offered as a mellifluous alternative. A mischievous student suggested "Calomel" for a newborn girl; the mother was unlikely to know that it was the name of a popular cathartic of the 1800s. A bold resident thought "Placenta" had possibilities (it designates the afterbirth of a delivery). "Brucella" has a crisp sound (it is a bacterium), so does "Filaria" (a blood parasite that causes elephantiasis), and "Alexia" sounds smart, but it means the inability to read.

Kindly nurses usually see to it that such suggestions are not adopted.

The pranksters may be forgiven; life surpasses them. A woman doctor named Euthanasia Meade practiced in California in the 1880s and a Placentia Whidden married a doctor in New Hampshire in the late 1820s. A mother named her newborn son "Pelvis" after she heard her doctors use the word repeatedly during her delivery which was made difficult by a bony deformity of her pelvis. She said she had never heard the word before, she liked the sound of it and thought it would make a fine name for her baby boy.

Another mother named an unexpected twin "Bonus" and was proud of her choice.

Some mothers cannot deliver their infants safely; a few cannot deliver them at all. A Cesarean operation may save the life of either or both the mother and the child. It was done in antiquity as the name suggests (though Julius Caesar was not born that way), but in those times the mother never survived.

Obstetricians enjoy doing Cesarean operations; it is not a difficult operation and the result is always spectacular — a baby! Dr. Kenneth Morgan described a contemporary experience.

"In performing a Cesarean section the obstetrician is often flattered by a considerable gallery of onlookers, mostly student nurses and medical students. The infant is extracted quickly and then the operation really begins, putting everything back the way it was — with the exception of the baby, of course. He is pleased that so many people are interested in watching him work; that is until he looks up. Lo and behold, the gallery has melted away. It is altogether deflating, but it's a fate that obstetricians have to face. You simply can't upstage a baby.

Unfortunately, not all babies receive the welcome that they deserve. Good-willed doctors have long been middlemen in the resolution of this dilemma. In the early 1800s Boston relatives brought unwanted newborns (usually delivered by midwives) to their doctors. The doctors found a place for the child and the child's keep was paid for through the doctor — identification was thereby avoided. Doctors lent their assistance out of friendship to their patients, and to prevent suffering, even death of the child. In the Boston practice of Dr. John C. Warren during this period, a baby in this category arrived almost daily at his office.

Dr. John Williams, professor of obstetrics at the Johns Hopkins Medical School through the first quarter of the 1900s, was moved by the human miseries that roil this aspect of life. He exerted himself to prevent the indiscretions and miscalculations of the vulnerable from bringing them useless, destructive obloquy.

When a young lady, widely known in Baltimore social circles told him that she was three months pregnant, a few weeks married and very worried. Dr. Williams calmed her fears — he would take care of it.

When the baby arrived. Dr. Williams told the assembled families that it was puny. He told the nurse to get a "preemie" crib (for underweight, prematurely born babies) and he cut and tore a preemie jacket to get the nine pound baby to fit into it. The baby was whisked away to the special preemie nursery and the families were told that it was so fragile that they would not be allowed to visit it — if it caught a single germ from them the result might be fatal.

After two weeks Dr. Williams announced that the baby had set a world record for growth. The child was now safe and healthy, not only ready to be visited, but could be taken home.

Dr. Williams cared for the pregnant wife of a parson on one occasion. She was forty years old and the parson was much worried — it was her first baby and at her age labor could be expected to be long and difficult.

Examination of the parson's wife diminished Dr. Williams' concerns; he found telltale signs of previous maternal experience. He assured the parson that she was in good health: things were quite likely to go well — but he approved of the parson's assertion that he would pray mightily. The baby was delivered after only two hours of labor. Dr. Williams told the parson that it was clear evidence of the power of prayer.

In the same era, Dr. Frederic Loomis, practicing in Los Angeles, encountered an unmarried young lady who was determined to keep her baby despite much advice to the contrary. She needed help to do it without ostracism and Dr. Loomis helped her.

There was a Salvation Army baby home nearby, and it

was always overcrowded. Dr. Loomis arranged for the young woman to keep boarder babies in her quarters temporarily, until there was room for them at the home. As soon as this practice was established — recognized by friends and neighbors and no longer of any interest to them — the doctor introduced the girl's own baby into the parade of boarder babies.

She took to it immediately and loved it so much that she "adopted" it.

When girls give what seem to be frivolous reasons for pregnancy it is impossible to say if they are exposing their ignorance, lost in superstition, or dissembling. Assertion that a pregnancy is due to bathing in a bathtub away from home is common. One young lady visited a married girlfriend on a weekend, forgot a nightgown, and borrowed one. She was adamant that her pregnancy was due to wearing the recent bride's nightgown.

A girl who was aghast at the announcement that she was pregnant said that if it was true it had to be due to the Holy Ghost. A whimsical doctor responded that while there was clearly a precedent for the claim, he was inclined to doubt that this was the second such incident. One very forthright girl reacted to a pregnancy determination with rage. When asked if she hadn't had intimate relations with men, she replied:

"Of course, but I wasn't married to any of them."

When the focus is on the failure to become pregnant folklore and superstition have provided remedies for ages and as an old one fades away a new one is certain to appear. In the 1970s nurses in a San Francisco hospital popularized a new way to assure conception. The method was to stand on one's head immediately after intercourse. Within a month of adopting this practice, seven nurses conceived.

5.

Education

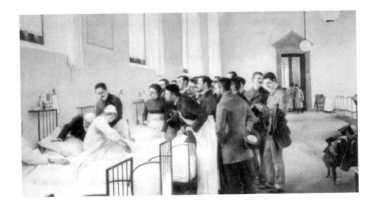

Completing the educational requirements of a modem medical school is a consuming affair. Students are often told on their first day of classes that when the sun goes down they will be behind in their work and learning and that they will never catch up. A medical student's private social life disappears.

Theron Clagett, subsequently an eminent surgeon at the Mayo Clinic, began his medical studies in 1929. He thought himself in love and engaged a young lady with his fraternity pin in the same year.

During his second year in school she returned the pin to him. She said that she was seeing him so infrequently that she really had no social life at all, and the prospect of continued neglect was too discouraging.

The prospect became equally discouraging for some of the medical students, especially the girls.

Dazed by the required intensity of medical study, some girls wondered; How did I get into this? What am I doing amidst the blood, bones, greasy muscles and foul odors when what I really like is history, art and music? They vented their misgivings in letters home; then they signed off with renewed determination:

"Now I have to get back to my studies."

One resolute girl arose at 4 a.m. each day to study. Her nonmedical roommate asked for a change of quarters; this study schedule was ruining her sleep.

An equally disciplined girl adapted to her studies by regulating her social life with precision. She allowed herself a bit of diversion on Saturday night, but it had to be carefully ordered: "First of all the escort had to be a man who would not be likely to involve the emotions too much. Otherwise some romantic entanglement might result and that would jeopardize the ability to concentrate on Sunday's studying. Second, he must be willing to terminate the evening by 11 p.m. so that I could get to bed early enough to be wide awake and ready to get back to work by 9 a.m. Sunday. Third, and most important, he must be smart enough to share my enthusiasm for the miracles of anatomy and chemistry and yet tactfully wean me away from the whole field of medicine for a few hours.... A few friends proved qualified on all counts."

What a very fortunate young lady to have such friends!

In the American Colonies most healers were self-appointed and self-educated. A few physicians educated in the medical schools of Europe drifted into the colonies; and after 1725 a small, but increasing number of young Americans sailed to Europe for a medical education — particularly to Edinburgh

— and returned to the colonies. Most young colonials who wished to become physicians did so by serving apprenticeships under doctors in one of these categories. The apprentice system represented the adoption of a practice that prevailed in Europe, and most American doctors were educated in apprenticeships until the time of the Civil War.

Before the Revolutionary War, apprentices served as long as seven years; after the war the period was usually two or three years. They paid one to two hundred dollars a year to their teachers. The apprentice read his teacher's books and watched him work. He learned to make pills, mix powders, and blend potions. He was also the house servant and the stable boy. Some doctors taught their apprentices and others ignored them.

An apprentice also learned to bleed, sweat, puke and purge the sick. These were the accepted treatments of the time. An apprentice with a little bit of medical learning was a character made for a comedy.

One such apprentice was sent to attend a lady suffering from a cough and some chest distress. He was directed to "cup her sternum." Cupping was blistering: a harsh, irritating substance was applied to the skin and confined under an inverted cup until it raised a large blister. It was painful, but the pain was thought to mollify any underlying disease.

The apprentice was competent at cupping, but he was less knowledgeable about anatomy. He did not know that the "sternum" was the breastbone; but he had worked on boats and he knew that the stem is the back end of a boat — surely the words were analogous. He applied his cups to the lady's buttocks and raised two very large and very distressing blisters there.

In 1765, America's first medical school was established at the College of Philadelphia, subsequently the University of Pennsylvania. A transformation of medical education began, but only two medical schools predate the Revolutionary War, and it was late in the nineteenth century before medical schools were widely established in our country. Philadelphia became our first great medical center.

In 1850 there were more than a thousand medical students in Philadelphia. They were a disorderly lot, so much so that respectable boarding houses rejected them. They could board only in a specific "Student District" of the city. Some students rented rooms elsewhere, but landlords were suspicious and if they found that they had a student tenant they were likely to move his belongings into the street while he was away. Medical students were troublesome.

In the student district a night watchman picked up and conveyed to their quarters any students who had over-indulged in spirits. He also bailed out any one who had been jailed, and he paid any unpaid debts or damage claims. The students settled with the watchman at the end of each month, and honor required a prompt and full settlement.

In classes the medical students chewed tobacco and spat the juice on the lecture room floors. A student wrote that there was so much tobacco on the floors that some young men wore rubbers to the lectures to protect their shoes.

The favorite classroom prank was "passing up." If a new-comer sat in the front row of the amphitheater — seats tacitly reserved for upper classmen — there would be angry calls from the back rows to "pass him up." This involved seizing the offender, hoisting him over head and passing him to the raised arms of the students in the second row who in turn quickly passed him on until he reached the top row of the amphitheater in a highly disheveled and discomfited state. Infractions of other unwritten rules and some singular habits or behavior were also discouraged by passing up.

A dean of the medical school at the University of Michigan recalled that only two limitations were placed on the pranks of medical students: they were not to assault any professors, and they must not bum down any college buildings.

The reputation of medical students and thus of medical schools was such that a few schools found it gainful to attract students on the grounds that they frowned on and discouraged student debauchery. In 1839 a brochure describing the Fairfield Medical College in western New York portrayed the school in very upright terms:

"The College is within eight miles of the Great Railroad from Albany to Utica and any medical student who is deterred from coming to the institution by the dread of riding over eight miles of country road had better choose some other profession than that of medicine.

"It is true that the village has only one tavern and no theatres except the anatomical, but it has three churches, a moral population, and good boarding houses. It is to be hoped that parents will think these advantages sufficient to counterbalance the wont of incentives to idleness and dissipation."

At Harvard in 1870 President Charles Eliot undertook to improve the quality and performance of the medical students. Among other things, he proposed written examinations. The professor of surgery, Dr. Henry Bigelow, objected on the grounds that more than half of the medical students could barely write. But Eliot persevered; he raised the admission requirements and strengthened the curriculum at Harvard. And in 1880 he wrote: "An American physician or surgeon may be and often is a coarse and uncultivated person, devoid of intellectual interests outside of his calling and quite unable to either speak or write his mother tongue with accuracy... In this university until 1870 the medical students were noticeably inferior in bearing, manners and discipline... they are now indistinguishable from other students."

This was not a miraculous transformation of young men; the less civilized element had been selectively eliminated.

In other schools improvement came very slowly. Dr. Arthur Hertzler studied at Northwestern University, in Chicago, in the 1800s and described the school: "Our school had two full-time men, the professor of chemistry and the janitor." In this period the professors were busy private practitioners. They lectured at the schools, but spent no other time with the students. Dr. Owen Stratton, who graduated from the Barnes Medical College in St. Louis in 1906, recalled that he had "never dressed a serious wound, never given a hypodermic injection and never been present at the birth of a baby."

Examinations were usually oral and sandwiched between or combined with other matters filling the professor's day. Dr. Edward Gifford described his final examination at the University of Pennsylvania in 1893. He was directed to appear at the home of Dr. William Pepper Jr., the professor of medicine. Dr. Pepper was an intellectual juggler who enjoyed performing several tasks simultaneously. When Gifford arrived, Dr. Pepper was eating, reading a newspaper and listening to a patient. Gifford offered to wait.

But Dr. Pepper brooked no delay; he reeled off a question and synchronized Gifford's examination into his act. Gifford described how he and the patient concluded one phase of the performance simultaneously — she with, "And my husband says he doesn't know what he'll do if I don't get some relief," and Gifford in another key with "and then the skin peels off the neck and chest and around the fingernails" — while Dr. Pepper ate his dinner and thumbed his newspaper.

Lecturing to a large group with whom the lecturer had no other contact had some pitfalls. In the 1880s biochemistry was a new subject, but already recognized to be as fundamental to medicine as anatomy.

A conscientious professor at the University of Michigan who lectured on the subject spoke slowly and deliberately to be sure that the students could follow him. On one occasion he was annoyed by a man in the front row who was obviously disinterested and making no effort to fellow the lecture. The professor focused on this man repeatedly during the lecture. His inattentiveness was distracting and by the end of the lecture the professor was furious.

He vented his wrath on the class. "This material is fundamental," he said. "You must master it. If you do not, it is useless for you to continue in school." To make the point

and further soothe himself he sought to shake up the obviously inattentive auditor. "You sir," he shouted. "Stand up
and let me ask you a few questions about the material we
covered today."

The object of this assault was so stricken that he was hardly
able to stand. He rose slowly and said, "Pardon me, doctor,
I'm not a member of this class. I have a letter of introduction
to you. I was waiting for the end of the lecture to present it
to you." The amphitheater exploded.

Professors were no better than fathers at predicting who
would succeed in medicine. In 1881 the professor of physiology at the University of Michigan examined students Franklin
Mall, William Mayo and Walter Courtney. He told each of
them after their examinations that they knew very little about
physiology and that they would not succeed in medicine. Mall
became a distinguished professor of anatomy at the Johns
Hopkins School of Medicine, Mayo became a peerless surgeon
and co-founder of the Mayo Clinic while Courtney became
chief surgeon for the Northern Pacific Railroad.

At the turn of the century two great changes occurred in
medicine. First, science was incorporated and laboratory studies became important; second, students were taken into the
hospitals for instruction at the bedside. Michigan established
the first university hospital in 1872.

Beginning in this period students were taught to observe
and scrutinize every aspect of a patient's appearance and
behavior for clues to the diagnosis of various diseases. They
learned to proceed the way Sherlock Holmes proceeded to
find the solution of a mystery. The Sherlock Holmes stories
were written by a physician, Conan Doyle, who created
Holmes in the image of one of his teachers who was a superb
medical investigator, i.e. observer.

At Harvard in 1905 Professor Harold Ernst honed his
students' powers of observation in an exercise that they would
never forget. He held up a glass of urine and itemized the
things that could be deduced about the donor from simple

observation: the color was amber, i.e., kidney function was good; the fluid was clear, i.e., there was no infection present, etc. Each of these things told the doctor something about the patient's health. The professor went on to say that urine ordinarily has a "sweetish taste" and to demonstrate it he put his forefinger into the glass of urine and then touched his tongue and lips.

"See if you agree," he said. "I'll pass the specimen around." Each student repeated the exercise, some manifesting a considerable squeamishness and distaste. When they finished, Professor Ernst said, "I observed each of you more carefully than you observed me. Notice that I put my forefinger into the urine, but my middle finger into my mouth." It was a widely used demonstration.

Students were taught that an educated sense of smell might detect important diagnostic clues even before a patient was examined. Patients with measles, typhoid, diphtheria and diabetes may emit distinctive odors. Patients with diabetes fared poorly at the turn of the nineteenth century; insulin had not yet been discovered and in the advanced stage of the disease diabetics tainted the air with the odor of acetone. Roger Lee , then a medical student at Harvard, told how he smelled a bottle of acetone daily for more than a year, preparing himself to make a brilliant diagnosis just by walking into a room where some patient without a diagnosis emitted the characteristic odor of diabetes. But the great day never came.

But it did come for Dr. Tom Cullen. As an intern Dr. Cullen was at one time in charge of a hospital ward with 144 cases of typhoid during an epidemic. A distinctive odor permeated the air of a typhoid ward, and Cullen never forgot it.

Many years later he walked into a hospital room and recognized the scent immediately. The patient's diagnosis was unknown; Dr. Cullen thought "typhoid" and ordered a laboratory test that would prove it. But the test was negative. Dr. Cullen visited the patient again —had the same reaction

— typhoid — and ordered the test repeated. It was repeated and again it was negative. Dr. Cullen visited the patient a third time — there was no mistaking the odor! He ordered the test once more and this time it was positive: the patient had typhoid.

Oliver Wendell Holmes once said that the nose — our sense of smell — recalls the past better than any other perception. Holmes would have loved this example. In 1950 an instructor at the University of Colorado School of Medicine called a student's attention to the "wet mouse" odor of a patient with diphtheria. It was an old and celebrated diagnostic clue, he said, an interesting historical oddity, one that the student would never encounter again because diphtheria was all but wiped out in the United States.

Seventeen years later the same student, now an Army doctor, came upon a sick child in Vietnam — the diagnosis was obscure. He recognized the wet mouse odor immediately and awed his colleagues with a prompt and correct diagnosis of diphtheria.

In the process of learning how to detect and recognize diseases, students have to master the use of the stethoscope. The stethoscope was invented in France in 1816; it came to the United States in the 1820s.

It led to great advances in the understanding of heart and lung disease.

Actually, an ear applied to the chest is equally effective and was the original way of detecting chest sounds, but it has some practical difficulties. In the 1940s a Harvard professor undertook to demonstrate the old-fashioned, direct method of listening to chest sounds to his students. He selected a female with long hair, parted her hair carefully and applied his ear to her back. His face took on a look of incredible dismay, matched by that of his student audience, as a head louse marched across the patient's skin just in front of the professor's eyes. He had demonstrated one of the practical problems that led to the invention of the stethoscope.

Students learn to use the stethoscope by examining each other; then they are permitted to examine selected patients to familiarize themselves with abnormal heart and lung sounds. If the patient is a female, the student must learn to displace the breasts without exposing the patient unnecessarily, and to do so with poise and detachment. The first few examinations are likely to be somewhat hesitant and clumsy.

At Bellevue Hospital in the 1940s, when a student made awkward attempts to listen to her heart, a forthright girl tested his equanimity to its limits. She said, "I don't usually let a guy get this far till after about three beers."

When the rectal examination is known to be the next day's topic, anticipatory apprehension is widespread among the students. A student wrote: "It was one thing to put a stethoscope on a friend's chest; it was quite another to stick a gloved and jellied finger up his rectum."

To be the object of this maneuver is even more unsettling. So when the instructor of one group proposed to do a demonstration in front of the class — before the students examined one another — and asked the class who would like to be first, there were no volunteers.

But a moment's calculation produced a volunteer. The student's reasoning was clear: This is bound to be easier than what a classmate will do to me.

Having learned what is normal, the students are assigned a hospital patient, told to make an examination, offer a diagnosis, and suggest a course of treatment. At this point, precision in language assumes a previously unappreciated significance. A third year student at Cornell University told other introduction to the subtleties of communication. Her first patient was an elderly, frail Chinese man. "I asked him to show me his teeth," she said.

Her patient was weak and quite ill; he got out of bed slowly to get at the drawer of his bedside table, drew his dentures from a dirty handkerchief and handed them to her for inspection. "I never asked about teeth again," she wrote. She asked her patients to open their mouths and she looked in.

When a diagnosis is considered, student doctors have a curious propensity to think of exotic diseases first; perhaps it is the striking names that bring exotic conditions to mind first. To counter this error, students are admonished: "When you hear hoofbeats, look first for horses, not zebras." And there is an alternative statement of the same principle for those who are more in tune with the language of Yogi Berra: "The common diseases are the ones encountered most commonly." And for the student who is inclined to guess or rely on laboratory tests there is the tongue-in-cheek counsel: "When all else fails, examine the patient."

After the examinations have been made, an instructor will often take a small group of students to revisit their patients. Each student presents his case in turn as the group moves about; the questions he asked, the answers he got, what he determined from his examination and finally his diagnosis. The patients' answers to questions necessarily require some transliteration when relayed to the medical group. Students commonly suffer shock and humiliation when at the end of an anxiety-ridden bedside presentation to an instructor and fellow students, the patient — who has listened to the medical rewording of his answers with some surprise — caps the event with, "I never said nothin' like that ever." Instructors assuage the student's embarrassment later: "Bear up," they say, "It happens all the time."

Of course some bedside presentations are prolonged and tedious. Students may be bored by their fellows' recitals, some stare out the window and others may focus on a nearby television screen. They may be so bored that even the patient in an adjacent bed is aware of it. One such observer commented that the students "looked like a bus load of tourists bored by the exhibits in the room."

Patient with unusual conditions that are particularly instructive may be asked to permit more than one student group to visit them in the company of instructors over several days.

Calculating students may solicit information from a group preceding them in order to enhance their performance if they happen to draw the same patient. A professor recalled that in his second year in medical school he was part of a group that examined a patient with a rare heart condition; his heart was on his right side rather than on the left. No student made the correct diagnosis.

The following day another student group visited the same bedside and was asked to examine the patient and offer their diagnoses. One young man made the remarkable diagnosis of a transposed heart. But no! Anticipating student collusion, instructors had moved the original patient to another part of the hospital.

As contact with patients is increased, the students must acquire the elementary skill of placing a needle in a vein to draw blood for laboratory tests or to administer fluids intravenously. This requires a bit of practice, and the tolerance of the subjects varies to the full extent of any scale.

A student on his first blood-drawing venture had two glass tubes to fill, but had only been able to fill one. His equally inexperienced student friend had visited a patient across the hall and failed to draw any blood. Both of them had irritated their subjects with multiple unproductive needle jabs.

What to do? They consulted in the hallway and agreed to exchange patients and try again. As the student with one tube of blood to his credit approached his new and distrustful patient, he was asked "Are you any better at this than the last doctor?" "Well, I've had a little more experience," the student replied. Later he mused, "I'm honest, I had drawn blood and he hadn't." This time they both succeeded.

Another student recalled an occasion when he failed to hit a vein on three successive attempts and he was perspiring. Worse, the patient had had many needles inserted previously without difficulties. He was a kindly man. He said, "Sit down, son, take a break. Get your nerve back. You can do it." They chatted for a while. Then the student tried again — and he succeeded. And the patient said, "Thank you!"

Some students noticed that when they appeared with their blood-drawing trays, patients held their breath until their beds were passed by.

As the students become engaged in patient care they are imbued with the principle of patient primacy: no patient need is to go unmet and what needs to be done is to be done promptly. This the core of good medicine; it is a very demanding commitment. Dr. Alton Ochsner, professor of surgery at the Tulane University School of Medicine in the 1930-1950 period, personified the principle of patient primacy and instilled it in his students. Early one morning on his hospital rounds, Ochsner listened as a student related the results of his examination of a patient admitted during the night while the student was on duty.

When the presentation ended, Ochsner asked for a bit of information that had been omitted; what did the rectal examination show?

The student explained that three patients had been admitted and assigned to him during the night.

He had done all of the examinations and all of the laboratory work; he had to get some sleep so he had deferred the rectal examinations until later. Dr. Ochsner caught the student by the lapels of his coat and drew him close, "My God, man," he said, making his point with extravagant hyperbole that would never be forgotten. "How could you sleep when you hadn't done a rectal?"

Most schools had quiz sessions in which a class gathered in an amphitheater and a professor reviewed a subject by presenting a patient and calling a student out of the group to come down and be grilled on all matters pertaining to the demonstrated disease. The students feared humiliation in front of their friends; they referred to the experience as being "thrown into the pit," or being "given over to the inquisitor."

At Johns Hopkins in the 1920s surgeon William Halstead conducted such clinics. Halstead was an intimidating man;

courteous, but remote and cold. At his clinics the students made up a pot of money, contributing twenty-five cents each, and gave it to the poor fellow who was called down and grilled.

At Tulane, Dr. Ochsner was a feared, aggressive examiner in amphitheater clinics. He flung his questions at the student and bore down on him sometimes actually backing the student across the floor of the amphitheater with his intimidating demeanor. One young man fainted dead away.

There were also weekly or monthly "Great" or "Grand" teaching conferences attended by all of the students and all of the faculty, in which a very complex diagnostic problem is presented. Faculty experts offer their opinions and the reasons for those opinions — for the benefit of the students — and the correct diagnosis is revealed only at the very end. The most famous of these conferences is the series once conducted regularly by Dr. Richard Cabot at the Peter Bent Brigham Hospital in Boston.

In the course of one of Dr. Cabot's conferences it was mentioned that the patient under discussion had "night sweats," and that night sweats suggested the presence of tuberculosis. Dr. Cabot did not think that there was any relationship between night sweats and tuberculosis. He said that many normal people perspire at night and he recalled his experience in France during World War I. He was often asked to treat French villagers, he said, and they all had night sweats because they slept with heavy woolen things on and kept the windows closed. Dr. Cabot turned toward neurosurgeon Harvey Cushing, who had also served in France, and asked, "Harvey, didn't you find that this was so when you were in France?"

And Cushing replied, "I can't answer that, Richard. I never slept with any of them." The students exploded and Dr. Cabot reddened to the top of his bald head.

When medicine was less hospital centered than it is today, students were sent out on medical as well as obstetrical house calls. Senior students made the calls; they were backed by experienced physicians whom the students engaged if they encountered something beyond their knowledge and experience.

Samuel Rosen, subsequently an accomplished ear surgeon, made such calls in Syracuse, N.Y., his home town, when he was a student at the Syracuse University College of Medicine in the 1920s.

On one occasion Rosen encountered an ill child who had a fever and a rash. His familiarity with rashes was nil; he could not make a diagnosis and he did not know how to proceed. But he had a resource unavailable to other students and he used it. His account is artful: "I did what any right-thinking boy would do; I called my mother and described the child's symptoms to her."

His mother was a better diagnostician. "He's got scarlet fever," she said — over the telephone — and she said it with total conviction.

Rosen returned to school and reported scarlet fever. Staff doctors were dispatched at once to confirm the diagnosis, which they did, and the house was quarantined. Dr. Rosen related how during the next three weeks he took a detour when he walked to school to look at the quarantine sign that proclaimed his diagnosis. "Scarlet Fever," it said. "And I diagnosed it," he wrote.

As with home deliveries, medical house calls produced many memorable encounters for the students. One student had gone to bed after a late supper of tinned sardines and potato salad. He was barely asleep when he was called to see a seventeen-year-old said to be very ill with abdominal cramps.

The boy was indeed in distress. He said that he had eaten wild cherries most of the afternoon.

With this clue, the student called for a basin, put two fingers down the boy's throat and up came the half-digested berries.

The sight and smell was so nauseating that the student "leaned over the basin and splashed the remains of my salad and sardines over the patient's berries." And he added, "We both felt better at once."

He was told later that the family regarded him as a hero because he was so sick himself when he came and cured their boy.

Students learn a great deal from auxiliary medical personnel: nurses, technicians, ambulance drivers, etc. Dr. Tom Rivers, director of the Rockefeller Institute Hospital through the 1940s, told how after two years of medical school he worked in a dispensary and was confronted with a patient who had a dislocated shoulder. The patient was brought in by ambulance and the ambulance driver volunteered the diagnosis. When Rivers seemed immobilized, the driver said, "You don't know how to set it do you?"

Rivers acknowledged his ignorance: "No, I've never seen one."

"I'll show you," the driver said. He put his foot against the patient's chest, pulled hard on the arm and the shoulder snapped into place.

Finally, graduation time arrives; medical students arrange some memorable parties in anticipation of the event. The graduation dinner of the Jefferson Medical College class of 1905 recalls the height of the medical student high-jinks era.

When the students arrived they found that the seats at the table were metal operating room chairs.

The tablecloths were surgical sheets and the napkins were diapers. Scalpels replaced the knives. Surgical gallbladder scoops served as spoons and special surgical clamps were the forks.

Each guest was given a surgical gown and a surgical cap. The table centerpieces were skulls and large bones. Cocktails were served in medicine glasses and wine in large test tubes.

It was said that "the most difficult moment," occurred when the waiters appeared with the serving dishes. Small urinals held the soup, bedpans brimmed with meat and vegetables and covered glass laboratory dishes, used to culture bacteria, displayed the fish. The account relates that a few students had to leave, but most were stout enough to enjoy the food.

At last, graduation day! One is a doctor, equipped for the future with a grand and special body of knowledge. But it proves to be only a beginning. The dean of the Harvard Medical School told a graduating class of the 1940s that he was sorry to let them know so belatedly that half of what they had been taught was surely false and then confessed that he wasn't even sure which half it was. Experience would provide the answer.

6.
Learning to Doctor

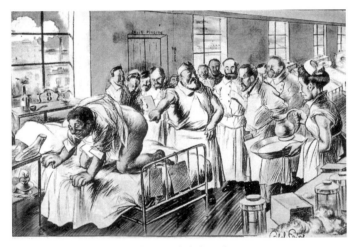

A beautiful fistula

Nurses usually make the first contributions to a young doctor's education when it is continued in a hospital after graduation from medical school. When I was an intern with just enough experience to find my way through the corridors of the hospital, I was called to see a patient who was complaining of abdominal distress. I found the proper ward and nurses station where I was welcomed by a smiling nurse who led me to the bedside of a thin, grizzled Afro-American holding his abdomen with both hands and writhing in pain.

I was cautious, I was a beginner; diagnosis is a wily game; I must be careful and systematic. As I stood at the bedside, the diagnostic possibilities rolled up on my mental screen: Appendicitis? Gallbladder disease? Intestinal obstruction? The rule that the most common things occur most commonly, came to mind.

Bladder problems are common, could this be a bladder problem?

To begin my examination, I asked, "Have you urinated today?"

"Whaaa...?"

I learned that he was hard of hearing. "Have you emptied your bladder today?" I asked. Perhaps "urinated," was too fancy a word, I thought —1 must speak plainly. "Whaaa...?"

We weren't communicating. The nurse shifted her feet slightly and I was afraid that it suggested some impatience with me. She was a pretty girl with glistening, black skin, a crisp white uniform, and a jaunty white cap. I glanced at her for support and her smile encouraged me to try again.

"Have you passed your water today?" I asked. I tried to keep my voice moderate; we were in a ward with nine other patients and most of them were sleeping.

"Whaaa...?"

How could he not understand? I was irritated, but the irritation was neutralized by a tinge of panic rising from my depths. What should I do next?

My comely, prim, supportive nurse came galvanized to my rescue. She pushed half in front of me, cupped her hands to her mouth, leaned over the old gentleman and shouted into his ear. "Pee! When was the last time you peed?" It brought every patient in the ward up to a sitting position.

"I can't," the old man said. "That's the trouble!"

The diagnosis was made. I was immensely grateful to the nurse for leading me, and much embarrassed that I needed to be led. But I had been given a lesson in communication that I would never forget.

Lessons from the nurses follow one day after another. Intern Pauline Stitt was called to do a spinal tap on a baby "about as big as a pint of ice cream." She had done spinal taps only on adults; she looked at the infant and didn't think she could do it. A nurse offered a pad of needles and Miss Stitt looked at them despondently.

The nurse smiled and said, "How would you use this needle?" She pointed to one on the sterile tray, but by no stretch the size needle that Miss Stitt would have chosen. She selected that needle and the spinal tap was accomplished swiftly.

Another intern told how he was suddenly faced with a patient requiring an emergency tracheotomy; the patient's breathing was obstructed and he was dying. An opening had to be made in his neck. The intern had never seen a tracheotomy. A brave and determined nurse offered to guide him through it and she did so step by step, successfully. The intern said he did the operation by remote control.

Of course, nurses were at the vital center for the acquisition of knowledge concerning odors.

An intern puzzled by a patient under his care and standing vacantly at the beside glanced at his nurse for reassurance. She responded, "Do you think he could have uremia?" she asked.

"Why would you think of that?" he asked.

"I think his breath smells of it," she said, and lab tests proved she was right.

He visited this patient daily during his days in the hospital to fix the odor of uremia in his mind. It was not widely known and was important. Some time later, in a train station, he was approached by a man asking for directions and noted that the man exhibited the distinctive odor of uremia. He gave out the directions and wrote a note for the man to take to a hospital; the note directed that the man be admitted to the hospital and treated for uremia. And later he received a note from the same man expressing his gratitude.

It is difficult to top a tale like that. But the same doctor encountered another similar situation.

This time he was rebuffed and the patient died.

The doctors and nurses who work side by side are often unknown to each other; work-mediated introductions are full of surprises. In the 1920s Dr. John Homans was a highly respected surgeon on the faculty of the Harvard Medical School. Homans had a marked lisp which was recorded on one occasion when he solicited the assistance of a young nurse in order to change a bandage on one of his patients.

"Thithter," he said, "go and get me a pair of thithorth — a therile one if you please."

The nurse disappeared for what seemed like an unduly long period and then returned to say. 'I'm thorry, thir, but I can't find a therile thithirth."

Homans was furious, "What the hell are you trying to do, imitate me?" "No thir," she said. "I lithp too."

A few nurses enjoy baiting the interns — in good humor. A pediatric nurse in a western hospital chewed up a "Baby Ruth" candy bar, spit a mouthful of it into a baby's diaper and brought it to her interns with an air of great concern. She remarked on the peculiarity of the diaper's content and implied that it might be of diagnostic significance. The interns were beginners; they had to agree. The nurse added that the contents had a peculiar smell and taste. Then she smelled it demonstratively and proceeded to put a sizable piece in her mouth as though she was tasting it again — while the interns turned green.

Accounts of the intern experience invariably report great anxiety, overwork (120-hour weeks were common and the range ran to twenty-four hours a day for fifty-one weeks of the year), lack of sleep and no pay. Surprisingly, the accounts usually end with a ringing statement to the effect that:

"It was by far the greatest year of my life."

Perhaps it was best described by the doctor who said he would not take a million dollars for the experience nor would he give a nickel to repeat it.

Mary Bates, who was the first female intern at the Cook

County Hospital in Chicago, described a common sequence: "The first six months were hell; the second six months were purgatory, the third six months were heaven; and when it came time to leave, I wept bitter tears."

Most interns were so busy that they seldom left the hospital. At Johns Hopkins in 1915, fellow interns told of one of their group who arrived with a new straw hat and did not have a chance to wear it again until he finished his internship.

The first task of the intern is to learn to deal with death. Euphemisms ease the disquiet until one becomes reconciled to it.

In one period at the Massachusetts General Hospital, the interns sang that no one died in their hospital; they went to Alien Street instead:

For in a well-run hospital
There's no such thing as death
There may be stoppage of the hearts and absence of breath
But no one dies!
No patient fries this disrespectful feat
He simply sighs, rolls up his eyes,
And goes to Alien Street.

The hospital morgue was on Alien Street.

There were also lesser things to adjust to. A young woman intern told how she learned to "wolf down a meal while discussing someone's innards."

A great goal of the intern is the acquisition of self-confidence. A little facetious arrogance aids the process. At one hospital a sign over the door to the intern's lounge read "Hero's Room." At another hospital the surgical interns complained loudly about being on call every other night. The trouble with the arrangement, they said, was that it caused them to miss half of the cases that came into the hospital.

A "can do" attitude prevails in a good intern: a good intern will find a way to fulfill every need.

Hospital x-ray departments commonly close at 5 p.m. A key is usually available to the interns on night duty, but inevitably it cannot be located when some intern needs the x-ray film of some patient. At the Boston City Hospital an indomitable intern took a huge metal x-ray department door off by its hinges one night to get the x-ray film he wanted.

The exploits of interns at the Boston City Hospital are justly famous. On one occasion a seventy-three-year-old lady came to the hospital for dizziness and a fluttery heart. Tests revealed a severe disturbance of heart rhythm, and hospitalization was advised.

She declined. Why? Because it was 3:30 p.m.; she had a chicken in the oven at home and it must come out at 5 p.m. for her husband's dinner. He was a cab driver.

The intern suggested that he call the cab company. The dispatcher could send her husband home to remove the chicken from the oven. But it wouldn't work. Her husband drove an independent cab without a radio. The intern suggested that he call the police. He could call it an emergency and the police could go to the house and remove the chicken from the oven. But it wouldn't work. A large, very mean German shepherd guarded the interior of the house and the police would have to kill the dog to get at the chicken.

The intern pocketed a packet of syringes and some emergency heart medicine — in case his patient took a turn for the worse. They would go to the apartment together, remove the chicken from the oven and return to the hospital. The intern had no car, so they would take a cab.

It was cold and snowing outside. The intern bundled up his patient and circled by the social worker's office to get some money for a cab. In the street there were no cabs in sight. When one appeared, the pair was ignored despite the intern's frantic signaling, and this was repeated several times. Finally the intern moved into the middle of the street. He would hijack a cab if necessary.

The next cab that appeared had no passengers, but the

driver didn't want any. He tried to circle around the intern, but the intern leaped onto the hood, pounding the metal with his fists and brought the cab to a halt. He threatened the driver who reluctantly accepted the fare and the lady was hustled into the cab. It was her husband's cab! The cabdriver-husband was sent home to attend the chicken and the intern escorted his patient back to the hospital.

In the hospital the pace is furious and the demands are rigorous. The credo that no patient's need is to go unmet — introduced to the medical students — is unwritten law for the interns. At Duke University, Dr. Eugene Stead was an exemplar of ideal medical dedication and discipline. On one of his morning rounds he listened to the description of a patient admitted during the night and discerned that a spinal fluid examination might throw some light on the diagnosis. "What did the spinal fluid show?" he asked.

The intern began the recitation commonly offered by students and sometimes offered by a new intern when something has been left undone: There was so much to do during the night, he had barely managed to get one hour of sleep.etc.

Dr. Stead was unmoved. "What you are telling me is that life is hard," he said. "What I want to know is what did the spinal fluid show?"

The standard insisted upon at a good institution is illustrated additionally in an anecdote related by surgeon Theron Clagett recalling his experiences as a resident in a hospital affiliated with the Mayo Clinic.

The chief of surgery required that every patient undergoing stomach surgery have his stomach emptied each morning thereafter via a stomach tube and that this be done for seven days. The resident was to do it and report it done for each patient when the chief surgeon made his rounds at 8 a.m.

One morning, one patient's stomach had not been emptied. The responsible underling explained that there had been fourteen stomachs to be emptied that morning. He had worked steadily since 4:30 a.m., but had not had time to do the last one before the 8 a.m. rounds. The chief surgeon's response was uncompromising: "Get up earlier," he said, "These stomachs must be emptied."

When these unwavering standards of care were inadvertently unmet there were some amusing scrambles for compliance. At the Johns Hopkins Hospital a conscientious young doctor was called to the emergency room to sew a bad cut sustained by a man who was intoxicated. The doctor completed the task and returned to his quarters and at that moment realized that he hadn't done a rectal examination. It was surely superfluous, but his examination was incomplete. He called the emergency room and was told that the patient was gone.

The doctor borrowed a car and drove to the saloon district of Baltimore. He walked down the center of the street calling his patient's name. Bystanders admonished him to be quiet, but then one bystander advised him to try Deacon's Saloon. When he did, the doctor found his patient asleep on a bench in the pool room. He picked up the patient, put him on a pool table, undid his belt, lowered his pants and did a rectal examination. Then he replaced his patient on the bench, went back to the hospital and made a note of the examination on the hospital record.

The interest and solicitude of the intern is quickly recognized by the patients. And because he is in semi-constant attendance, the intern is often perceived as the doctor. The relationship that develops is exemplified in the tale about a nationally famous consultant who came some distance at special request to examine a patient and then recommended an operation. The patient deferred his decision. He said he wanted to talk it over with *his* doctor first — *his* doctor turned out to be the intern.

The heavy workload was tolerated goodnaturedly. It was difficult, but it was gratifying.

Some interns described themselves as "smiley tired." Hospital personnel helped them and humored them.

A female telephone operator at one Boston hospital made an early morning wake-up call to the intern's quarters and regularly told whoever answered to, "Get that woman out of your bed!"

Fatigue had some amusing consequences. At the Boston City Hospital an exhausted intern slipped out of the hospital to a restaurant a few doors away to treat himself to a steak. He fell asleep over his dinner and was awakened by a waiter who assured him that he had eaten his steak and presented him a bill for $5.95 to prove it. The intern departed, still hungry, not really sure that he had eaten a steak and much disappointed that he had no recollection of the pleasure he had so eagerly anticipated.

Another Boston intern was working thirteen-hour shifts, seven days a week when he was invited to take a break at Martha's Vineyard for a weekend. To accumulate the necessary free time he worked — along with his usual shift — an additional Tuesday night, all of Thursday night and most of Friday night. He arrived at his hostess' home Saturday afternoon, fell asleep and was awakened on Sunday afternoon just in time to make it back to Boston.

The penury — no pay — could be combatted in various ways, most commonly by giving blood for patients who needed transfusions. In the 1960s interns at Bellevue Hospital in New York thought themselves affluent. They received room and board and uniforms, and they could donate blood two or three times a month for twenty-five dollars a pint. And by law a blood donor was entitled to a pint of whisky after each transfusion. The whisky was quite saleable and the interns were not above writing prescriptions for whisky which were also saleable.

At some hospitals research projects created additional opportunities for interns to earn some money: they were readily available subjects for experiments. The cure for pernicious anemia was discovered at the Boston City Hospital in 1926. The cause was found to be a deficiency in the secretions — the gastric juice — of the stomach. When the research leading to this discovery was in progress, the interns sold their gastric juice for study: two dollars for half a cup. They had to swallow a stomach tube and have the juice siphoned out, but for two dollars that was no deterrent.

When hospital training programs for doctors (internships) were first established — during the transition from the nineteenth to the twentieth century — interns were forbidden to marry. The best teaching hospitals would not appoint a medical school graduate who was married, and they threatened to drop any intern who did marry. This was true until World War II when the scarcity of interns abolished the bias.

In 1914 a Boston intern at the Peter Bent Brigham Hospital was engaged and wanted to marry. He discussed it with his superior who in this instance was neurosurgeon Dr. Harvey Cushing. Cushing was negative: "Can't she wait?" he asked, "My wife waited for me for eight years." Another of Cushing's trainees married without consulting or informing him. When he was confronted in a meeting with Cushing and members of his staff, he said, "I promise I won't do it again." Everyone laughed heartily — except Cushing — but he didn't pursue the matter; it had been turned into comedy.

Through the 1920s trainees under Cushing regarded any association of their names with marriage, even a hint of it, as very dangerous. One who was unable to leave the hospital for long periods arranged for the hospital admitting desk to page him and inform him when his "sister" arrived. He met his fiancee in an anteroom two to three times weekly in the evening. They held hands and shared the treats she brought while he dictated case notes until 1 or 2 a.m.

In the same period, when Johns Hopkins selected one group of interns they considered a young man who had stellar academic record and an engaging demeanor. But there was a problem: he was married. He was told that he would be accepted if he made arrangements for his wife to live at least fifty miles from Baltimore.

Elsewhere an intern proposed marriage after a four-month courtship despite anticipated disapproval. He told his medical girl friend that they either had to get married or stop seeing each other — it was too exhausting. Another intern married and hid his wife in a nearby motel.

Dr. Richard Cattell, later a principal surgeon at the Lahey Clinic in Boston, devised a unique solution to the marriage problem. He married while he was a resident in 1925. He had no money for the venture. He sold blood to pay for the wedding ring and married a girl who shared an apartment with a friend. Dr. Cattell moved into the apartment and made it a menage a trois. It worked because he was only there every third night.

Hospital romances conducted on the premises have received a great deal of attention — and long before the sitcom era. The ingenuity and audacity with which some of these affairs were conducted probably cannot be overdrawn, but the implied frequency is surely exaggerated. Concerns about this matter are the material for more comedy. When John Shaw Billings, the great hospital planner of the era, planned the Johns Hopkins Hospital — opened in 1889 — he proposed that the hospital have only small closets. He wrote: "If a female nurse is a properly organized and healthy woman, she will certainly at times be subject to strong temptation under which occasionally one will fall, and this occurs in all hospitals when women are employed. Something may be done, however, to remove opportunities and I believe that the construction proposed (the elimination of all large closets Ed.) affects this as far as it is worth while to attempt it."

Perhaps this construction did reduce trysting in the closets, but it did not eliminate it. Another Dr. Billings, the planner's son, was subsequently a trainee at the hospital and told how he and the nurse who later became his wife sometimes met in one of the small closets.

In many hospitals through the first quarter of the twentieth century, interns were forbidden to date nurses. At the

Newark City Hospital in 1905, conversation between interns and nurses was forbidden inside and outside of the hospital except that having to do with hospital duties. Of course, such absurdities were ignored. But they created material for more comedy. At the Newark hospital, the nursing supervisor was the enforcer, but when she moved about the hospital a system of rattling ropes in the dumb-waiters kept everyone informed of exactly where she was at all times.

An intern was usually selected to respond to calls from the dormitory associated with the hospital's nursing school. It was a coveted assignment — a great opportunity to meet nurses. At the Cook County Hospital, this intern was referred to by his fellows as the "Court Physician."

Professional appearances suffered a severe decline among interns during the 1960s when some free spirits made long hair and blue jeans their signature. But it recovered. In the '70s an incoming intern group was lectured to "make sure you look like you are here to cure disease and not to spread it."

Interns were likely to be the doctors best informed about new treatments and the most eager to try them out. New treatments lead to new and sometimes unexpected results. In the 1940s an ether-in-oil enema was alleged to be a new effective treatment for asthma. A Boston intern encountered a patient in the throes of an asthmatic attack and proved that the method could be effective in a manner that had not been previously appreciated. The appropriate enema was administered and the patient expelled it in the bathroom. Then he dropped his cigarette into the toilet. The ether exploded and sent him running down the hallway completely relieved of his asthma by the surge of his own adrenalin. "My God, Doc," he said. "I exploded."

Some heroic exertions also produced unanticipated results. One intern initiated an alarm for an emergency heart team to come to his ward and he assisted in an attempted cardiac resuscitation. It was a violent affair, conducted on the floor, including surgical entry into the patient's chest for heart massage — and it failed. Half of the patients on the ward promptly signed out of the hospital.

An innovative intern could convert some medical procedures into diverting amusements for himself and his patients. A Boston intern undertook to entertain the Irish on St. Patrick's Day. In evening of the day before St. Patrick's Day he ordered a small dose of a harmless blue dye — sometimes used as a urinary antiseptic — for every Irishman on his ward. The dye turns the urine green. On the morning of St. Patrick's Day, to their great delight, every Irishman passed green urine and the non-Irish did not.

When the interns changed from one hospital section to another, usually every three months, they held "change parties." Alcohol for these parties could be abstracted from the stocks in the laboratories — the interns had the keys at night. If the laboratories were too strict with their accounting, there was an alternative method. The interns could order an evening highball for each of a host of patients, and then connive with the nurses to see that they were not delivered — the alcohol was accumulated for the party.

Rotation through the hospital services includes a stint in the emergency room. An emergency room prepares an intern for anything he is likely to see in the future. It is commonly referred to as the "pit," or the "combat zone." The intern on duty there is often labeled as either a "gate," or a "sieve," meaning that he controls hospital admissions effectively or that he allows entirely too many people to enter the hospital. A sieve in an emergency room can easily overwhelm the doctors on the floors above.

An emergency room has a drollery of its own. A whimsical physician collected some of the scenes he encountered there. A distraught mother brought her child in because he drank the dog's milk — from the dog's nipples she added. Another had placed an extruded baby tooth under her child's pillow. It was now lodged in the child's right ear. And another mother was very concerned about a piece of bologna string which was hanging from her baby's anus.

Mothers make telephone inquiries to emergency rooms. One said, "Hello, I would like to schedule an emergency." Another called to say, "My baby can't breathe. What time can I bring her in?" And among the nighttime encounters there was a man who came in at 4 a.m. because he had had two bowel movements on the prior day instead of his usual one.

To deal with these and many less amusing but equally minor troubles, emergency rooms pursue the only course possible, epitomized in the dictum, "Treat 'em and Street 'em."

An unwary Boston intern was the principal player in one emergency room comedy. He attended a party at the apartment of newlyweds where highballs were served in breakfast glasses because the couple had yet to acquire any fine glassware. The guests had various troubles after leaving. The intern had a ticket to a concert at Symphony Hall and he got there, but he passed out in the men's room. A rescue squad delivered him to his own emergency room where he was received with a mixture of raised eyebrows and hilarity.

His reception was restrained. In another similar instance, an intern who overindulged in spirits and was brought to his own emergency room in something between somnolence and unconsciousness, and his colleagues were mischievous as well as amused. The intern awakened to find himself immobilized in a plaster cast that extended from head to foot and with a catheter dangling from his bladder.

Boston City Hospital interns amused newcomers for years by recalling the only white man ever admitted through the emergency room as a black. He was an alcoholic who lived among the ashes from an old boiler in an abandoned building when he was brought in. After a midnight bath, his designation was hastily changed to white.

The most remarkable patrons of the emergency rooms are the "simulators." They are a bizarre group of people who perfect an ability to simulate the symptoms of almost any known disease. They do it expertly. They come to the hospital emergency rooms pretending to be ill and demanding immediate treatment. They solicit test procedures of every variety, and even major operations.

Most of them want room and board, a day or two in the hospital after which they leave abruptly, expressing great disapproval of their treatment no matter what it was. Some want narcotics or sleeping pills, but a few want surgery and will skillfully mislead doctors into any variety of major operation. They bear the scars of operations on the appendix, the gall bladder, the kidney, and even the brain. Some select a busy street corner where they can feign collapse and be sure that a crowd will gather immediately, a policeman will appear and an ambulance will arrive promptly to rush them to a hospital.

This curious behavior is called the "Munchausen Syndrome." It was named for a German baron of the eighteenth century who was widely known as a teller of tall tales. Dr. William Bean, of the University of Iowa described this disquieting obsession in verse:

> *Baron Munchausen, a fabulous liar*
> *The syndrome's eponym did inspire*
> *Hospital haunters, doctor deceivers*
> *Their acting confounds even non-believers*
> *Whence does he come and what does he seek?*
> *They seem to thrive and gain elation*
> *From many a needless operation*
> *Often departing before they heal*
> *Then into another hospital they reel.*

This group includes people who bleed themselves to life-threatening anemias, lacerate their colon with a knitting needle to provoke intestinal bleeding, draw blood and swallow it in order to vomit it and pass blood in their stools and inject multiple materials under their skin to create infections. There is a group who abuse their own children to create medical conditions that require a doctor's care; this is known as the "Munchausen Syndrome by Proxy." And computer networks have created a new dimension, Munchausen types who join support groups and tell false tales of illness. They get the information they need from the same computers.

Emergency room personnel become very wary, but they are repeatedly nonplussed. When a drunken man presented himself at a Boston emergency room on a cold winter night and said that he had been run over by a truck, he was regarded with amused disbelief: this was surely a sham. But when his shirt was removed tire tracks stood out clearly on his chest. And in Philadelphia a man came into an emergency room on a bitter night presenting a lacerated hand. He said he had been bitten by an elephant — highly unlikely. But he was sober and it turned out that he had been feeding some circus elephants in winter quarters not far from the hospital.

As they rotate between medical sections, surgical wards, the emergency room and the obstetrical services of their hospitals, the interns teach the students and learn from the residents who are the previous year's interns. The terms intern and internship were dropped in 1975. The equivalent person has since then been designated the first-year resident. The teaching process is governed by the precept, "See one, do one, teach one." Irreverent residents modify it to, "See one, screw one, teach one."

New sets of mnemonics are useful in the hospital; they deal with diagnosis rather than anatomy.

The "Five Fs" was a widely used mnemonic that calls to mind the features lending support to a diagnosis of gall bladder disease. It is impressed on memory by a story of an intern examining a lady in a hospital clinic.

He suspected that she had gall bladder disease and he reviewed the "Five Fs" in his mind: she was fat, a female, she was fertile (she had several children), and she was forty. He was striving to recall the fifth "F" when he heard a sharp report and a fetid odor filled the examination cubicle. "Ah, yes," he thought, "That's it. The fifth "F" — flatulence!"

Recent studies have indicated that the "Five Fs" are of little or no significance, but the mnemonic has a place in history and the story is a gem in the record of medical humor.

Ambitious residents are alert for opportunities to advance medical knowledge: they are eager to become medical authors. Doctors at the University of Pittsburgh were delighted when a distressed child in their emergency room was found to have a cockroach in each ear. A cockroach in one is common enough in any large city emergency room, but a cockroach in each ear is a rare thing. The doctors in Pittsburgh "recognized immediately that fate had granted us the opportunity for an elegant, comparative therapeutic trial."

It is difficult to completely remove a live roach from a child's ear; instrumental pulling and prying risks injury to the inner ear. Doctors have debated the value of two alternative methods for years. Some fill the ear with mineral oil which kills the roach, and then remove it through an ear scope. Others fill the ear with lidocaine, a local anesthetic, which may force the roach to leave. Here was an opportunity for a decisive experiment.

The Pittsburgh doctors put mineral oil in one ear. The roach succumbed "after a valiant struggle, but required considerable dexterity for removal." When a lidocaine spray was directed into the other ear, the occupant exited "at a convulsive rate of speed and raced across the floor." The conclusion was clear, it was publishable, it resolved " a problem that has bugged mankind throughout recorded history."

Another emergency room that had recommended putting oil in the ear in response to a telephone call received a second call from the same party and the query, "Which ear?"

Residents take their responsibilities so seriously that it is easy for them to attribute too much significance to their acts. In October 1965 a Boston resident intent on recording an electrocardiogram on one of his patients could not find a working electrical outlet near his patient's bed. He finally located one at a distance and ran an electrical cord down the hall to activate his heart machine.

As he plugged in the cord, the entire hospital went dark. He was dismayed — dispirited that he should be the one responsible for a hospital collapse of this magnitude. As he wondered what to do first he heard on a portable radio that the blackout extended from the Canadian border to New York City. My God, he thought, what have I done? It was the great Northeastern regional power failure.

As the resident doctors work in the various divisions of their hospitals, they consider the kind of doctor they might like to be. One thought that he might like to an obstetrician. It was nice, he observed, to send a patient home with something besides a bill. A young woman resident also liked obstetrics. She liked it because both the doctors and the patients seemed to be happy most of the time. But another young woman was turned away. Caring for two patients in one body is too much, she said.

A radiologist told the young doctors that looking at pictures of patients was more pleasant and rewarding than looking at people. A dermatologist seemed very pleased with his specialty. His patents didn't die and they never seemed to get well.

A surgeon confided that surgery was a great specialty; you didn't have to talk to patients. The resident he spoke to said that he didn't mind talking, but that he had noticed that adults lie a great deal to their doctors. Children told the truth, he said, even while their mothers were telling them to shut up. Therefore, pediatrics might be a good specialty. And one resident was advised by his fellows that he had a dirty mind — he should be a psychoanalyst.

Jocelyn Elders, who became surgeon general of the United States, said that she liked every specialty division of the hospital she worked in as a resident: "Every service I went on, that's what I wanted to be."

7.
Waiting For Patients

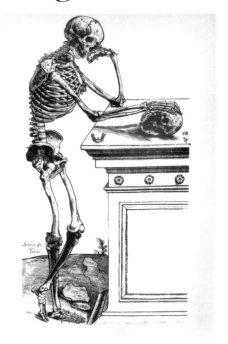

Very likely no doctor ever opened an office and failed to attract any patients. But it is equally likely that every young doctor sitting in his newly opened office has feared that it might happen to him.

Dr. Benjamin Rush, the Philadelphia physician-patriot of the Revolutionary War era, advised his apprentices that a doctor's practice increased more rapidly if he was regular in his attendance at church.

"Worship with the Mohammadans rather than stay home

on Sundays," Rush said.

Young doctors followed Dr. Rush's advice. But some devised ways of acquiring the religious aura for a minimal investment of time. They arranged to be called from church shortly after they arrived. They paid a boy to appear at the church and say that the doctor was needed immediately.

During the week, the new doctors sat in their offices and waited. While they waited, they read.

Dr. Samuel Gross opened an office in Philadelphia in 1826 after graduating from Jefferson Medical College.

He did a great deal of reading. In less than a year, he translated a textbook of anatomy, a manual of obstetrics, and a textbook of surgery from French into English, and a monograph on typhus fever from German into English. After eighteen months of enough leisure to complete this work — interrupted by very few patients — Dr. Gross moved to Easton, Pennsylvania.

Dr. Arthur Hertzler explained the basis for the often heard jokes about the magazines in doctors' waiting rooms being so much out of date. It was because the doctor had plenty of time to read and he had all of the current issues in his private office. A doctor's wife offered an alternative explanation. She said that she always missed some installments of serial stories because patients made off with the current issues.

The office of a nineteenth century doctor usually consisted of two rooms. One served as a waiting room and the other as a combined office-treatment room. In the Midwestern settlements, one room was often the complete office, serving both as a waiting room and a treatment room. This arrangement, in which patients watched the treatment of persons who preceded them, might severely unnerve some of those who were waiting.

Until he could afford additional quarters, a young doctor might sleep in his waiting room. Dr. Howard Kelly, later one of the "Famous Four" professors at Johns Hopkins Hospital, opened his first practice from two rooms in Philadelphia in

1883. He slept on the sofa in his waiting room at night. Kelly attached one end of a string to one of his big toes and dangled the other end of the string out of a window. Patients were to pull on the string if they wanted him at night.

Funds for the rent and the furnishings of an office required some local credit confidence or investor anticipation. Dr. William Rohlftold told how he managed it in Hampton, Iowa, in 1891. He had no funds, but he rented two rooms over a drugstore. The druggist banked on some prescriptions as security. But the local furniture dealer hesitated to supply the necessary furnishings on credit.

It occurred to Dr. Rohlftold to ask the furniture dealer if he was perchance also an undertaker, a common combination. He was. "I reminded him that I was young and inexperienced.. He saw the point and agreed to furnish the office."

Dr. Thomas Salmon graduated from the Albany Medical College in New York in 1899. He bought an office and a medical practice from a doctor who was retiring. The purchase included a case of surgical instruments that were somewhat rusty and dated, but Dr. Salmon thought that if he polished them up and displayed them they would add prestige to the appearance of his office. They had been exhibited in a cabinet for about a year when Dr. Salmon discovered that they were veterinary instruments.

Location is of great importance when a doctor opens an office. In Chicago in 1909, Dr. Paul Magnusen was ready to open an office for the practice of orthopedics. A survey of the city convinced him that the busiest place in town was at the entrance to the famous Chicago Stockyards. He found two rooms over a saloon near the stockyard entrance, one room to live in and one for an office. He expected to see men injured in the stockyards and he could also expect a few from the saloon. There was an additional boon. The bartender agreed to take his telephone calls when he was out.

When Dr. Milton Slocum chose to open a practice in Manhattan in the early 1930s, he selected a street crossing the central portion of the island — 56th Street — as the general locale. Then his wife scouted the street that crossed 56th and counted the pedestrians on them to ascertain which ones carried the most foot traffic. When she had narrowed the focus, she determined which side of each street was the more heavily traveled, and when she had settled on the busiest street and the busiest side, she searched for and found street-level rooms where a window sign would be easily seen and likely to attract patients.

Streets may have other significance and some are "Doctor Streets." One doctor told how when he moved his office just a few blocks to a street of high medical repute he received dozens of congratulatory messages. He was moving up.

The atmosphere surrounding an office is also important and it may require continued attention. In Philadelphia, a doctor was upset when a mortician more than once parked his hearse in front of the doctor's office when he called to pick up a death certificate. The doctor told him to please park elsewhere — the farther away the better.

Inevitably some advice to young doctors is conflicting. One told how a friend advised him to remove the well-filled bookshelves from his office. Doctors are supposed to know, the friend said, and not have to consult books. It would have a bad effect on patients. One young woman doctor was of a like mind. She kept two medical textbooks in a nearby lavatory where she could consult them. But another friend was of a different mind. He told of a visit to another doctor's office and added that there wasn't a book in sight, "so he can't know much."

Miscellaneous interested parties try to give the new doctor's practice a boost. A doctor who opened a practice in Philadelphia and was attracting only an occasional patient received a call from a medical friend who seemed alarmed: "Don't you know that it is unethical to advertise?" he said. It was considered unethical at that time.. The doctor was astonished and puzzled — he hadn't advertised.

He learned of an advertisement in a Jewish newspaper that credited him with great and unusual medical skills. His landlady had become concerned about his ability to pay the rent and thought that the ad might benefit both of them.

The best way for a young doctor to gain patients is to cure one of the community's chronically-ill persons, preferably the one that all of the doctors in the area have treated and failed to cure. But any strikingly successful case will do, even if the success is fortuitous. Dr. Lewis Thomas, the essayist, told how his father's practice was increased. His father was young and unknown in Flushing, Long Island, when a patient came to him complaining of blood in his urine. Examination of the patient and a few office tests revealed nothing. To buy time in which to read up on the matter, Dr. Thomas gave his patient some iron pills — good for anemia — and told him to come back in four days.

The patient returned in four days carrying a flask of crystal-clear urine and he was delighted. The word spread quickly. Dr. Thomas was even said to possess gifts beyond his own knowledge because he insisted that the pills he had given had nothing to do with the improvement. The patient doubtless had a kidney stone which passed silently, as they often do. For Dr. Thomas it was a lodestone. It attracted patients.

Other fortuitous events sometimes generate a practice for a waiting doctor. In 1846 a well-educated physician put up his shingle in Bennington, Michigan. He waited from May to September without seeing a single patient. Then an epidemic swept through the area and he was busy continuously making calls and making himself known to every family in the surrounding countryside.

A Texas doctor inadvertently created his own timely event. He graduated from Tulane University in 1885 and opened a practice in Comanche, Texas. He had no funds and the prospect for acquiring any soon was very dim. But on the third day after his arrival, his children came down with the measles that quickly spread to the whole community and kept him very busy.

But most doctors do not acquire patients quickly by virtue of a dramatic cure or a timely plague. One of our early women doctors opened a practice in San Francisco in 1900 and described some of the miscellaneous reasons why patients came to her office. A woman selected her for maternity care because the doctor she chose in her previous pregnancy had put a medicine bottle down on her nice mahogany dining table and left a mark that she had never been able to remove.

Another woman had four boys and wanted a girl. She thought that pregnancy management by a female physician might produce the desired result. It was a boy.

And a husband brought his wife in because he thought that the charge by a woman doctor would be less. When he was told that the fee would not be less, he was decently gracious. He said, "Oh well, I'll take you anyway. You probably need the money more than the men do."

One doctor's heart was warmed by his welcome to a new community. The maid of a rich woman came with a fine pheasant. The doctor's wife cooked the pheasant and they greatly enjoyed the dinner.

Then came a telephone call from the town's established physician: "I believe you have my pheasant."

Oliver Wendell Holmes warned young doctors that the public likes its doctors "moldy." Of course Holmes couldn't anticipate medical advertising. Before advertising became acceptable there were only a few things a young doctor could do. The wife of a doctor who opened a home office in the 1920s described some of them. When they needed a loaf of bread, he grabbed his medical bag and rushed out of the door. Neighbors might notice and think he was busy. And when he needed a haircut, he carried his medical bag and rushed out of the door. Someone might notice and think he was busy. But most of the time, he just waited.

There were some individualized exceptions. Youthfulness could be combated. A particularly youthful looking doctor bought himself a pair of horn-rimmed glasses with clear lenses and wore them continuously. It changed his image. And another doctor gave all of the patients he had appointments on the same day at the same time so that the waiting room would be full and it would appear that he was very busy.

Community service offers a doctor some opportunities to make himself known. These activities are gratifying. Sometimes they are unexpectedly amusing. When surgeon Frederick Christopher was establishing a practice in the 1920s, he was asked to address a large group of Girl Scouts in Chicago. He was pleased. He talked to them about first aid for various injuries, about controlling bleeding and about splints for broken bones. At the end of his talk he offered to answer questions and was disappointed by the dead silence. Finally a girl arose with a question. Dr. Christopher was delighted. Perhaps it would draw out other children. "Yes, Miss," he said. "What is your question?" And with the utmost seriousness, the girl asked, "Could you tell me what makes my grandmother have so much gas?"

In the same period, Dr. S.E. Gibbs attended church socials to make himself known to his community. He told of meeting an elderly lady who related a long string of ailments, some of her husband's maladies and a few medical problems of their grandchildren. He wrote, "Of course, I sympathized with her, but offered no advice." He heard later that she liked him personally, "but would not care to employ a doctor who takes so little interest in his patients."

For obvious reasons, medical colleagues are not usually helpful when a new doctor opens an office.

But when Dr. John DaCosta opened his practice in Philadelphia in the late 1880s, he was impressed by the generosity of his colleagues; it seemed that most of them had promptly directed one or two patients to him.

But Dr. DaCosta's regard for his fellow physicians crumbled quickly. To the last one, these patients turned out to be difficult, censorious of doctors and addicted to demanding medical attention during the nocturnal hours. Alcohol played a large role in their medical problems, they lived "at the jumping off fringes" of the town, and it never occurred to any of them to pay a bill.

First patients are likely to be memorable. Dr. DaCosta remembered his first patient very well. His first patient stole his only umbrella out of the waiting room.

And a doctor who opened an office in New York City in the 1950s recalled that his first patient, a man with pain in his abdomen, walked in before the office examination table arrived. How to examine the patient? There were two choices: on the floor or on the office desk — it was embarrassing. The doctor cleared the top of his desk and asked the patient to loosen his trousers and to lie down on it. "Fortunately he was not tall and just about fit."

To mollify his patient, the doctor spoke of battlefield conditions, babies born in automobiles, and surgery performed on kitchen tables as he examined his patient. But he worried about what the man was thinking, probably, "How do I get out of here?" The doctor wrote a prescription for the patient and asked him to telephone in two days. Of course, he never saw the patient again.

Dr. Robert Goldyn, who opened an office for plastic surgery in Boston in 1963 also recalled his first patient. Less than two hours after he opened his door, an elderly gentleman walked in. Both Dr. Goldyn and his secretary were ecstatic. How had he heard of Dr. Goldyn, they asked. He hadn't. He didn't see well, he was looking for his ophthalmologist and had wandered into the wrong office.

A young doctor in Detroit responded quickly when he was asked to see a sick lady at home. He was shown into her bedroom by her husband who then waited outside. Very shortly the doctor came to the door and asked for a short piece of wire with a hook on the end. After five minutes the doctor appeared again and asked for a pliers, and after another five minutes he reappeared and asked for a small hammer.

The husband supplied all of these things, but he was puzzled and beginning to be concerned. "Please tell me what is wrong with my wife?" he asked. "I don't know," the young doctor replied. "I haven't been able to get my bag open."

Losing one's first patient could be ruinous. Prospective patients were alarmed and driven away. Dr. Charles Meigs, later a professor of obstetrics at the Jefferson Medical College in Philadelphia, began his medical career in Augusta, Georgia, in 1816. His first patient, a prominent person in the community, died of a fever. It was customary at that time for doctors to walk in funeral processions, often at the head of the parade. Meigs was dismayed. He thought he would rather be flogged. He was sure that every eye would be focused on him and that all of the conversation would be about his failure. But he walked and to his astonishment his appearance introduced him to a great many people who did not know of him and his practice flourished.

Dr. Benjamin Dudley found it hard to sit and wait. He opened an office in Lexington, Kentucky, in 1806 and practiced patiently for two years. At the end of that time he was still not making a living. Dr. Dudley took some aggressive remedial action. He bought a flatboat, loaded it with produce and floated down river to New Orleans. He sold his produce and invested the proceeds in flour. He shipped the flour to Lisbon, Portugal, accompanied it across the ocean and disposed of it for a good profit. Then he visited Paris and London to learn all he could about surgery.

Dudley then returned to Lexington where his new knowledge and European aura brought him prompt success. He created the Transylvania Medical College in Lexington, the first medical school west of the Alleghenies.

Throughout the nineteenth century it was not unusual for a doctor to move from village to village, failing to thrive in one and moving on to try again in another. One of our early female doctors set out to practice in a small town where several other doctors had failed and departed. She was having limited success and she sensed that she also was expected to be transitory. She bought a lot in the local cemetery to convey a contrary message and she stayed.

There were too many doctors in the United States because there were no educational requirements for doctors. Anyone who wished to do so could assume the title. In 1831, the *Boston Medical and Surgical Journal* recognized the over supply of doctors and the low level of their income: "A man is compelled to labor patiently for many years in a city before he can command his daily bread in exchange for prescriptions." In 1832, a steamboat exploded on the Connecticut River and a doctor drowned in the accident. The news set off a stampede of doctors to replace him.

When the Midwest was being settled it was necessary to teach school or find some other second occupation if one practiced medicine. In Indiana there were so many doctors that one who wished to take a vacation back East did not dare to do so. He wrote that another doctor would replace him immediately and remain permanently — if he departed for even a brief period.

In the commencement address to the medical graduates at Yale in 1841, the speaker reiterated the same theme. He said that medical practice offered the "possibility of self-support, but little else." Many doctors abandoned medicine. Moses Appleton, a Harvard graduate who practiced in Waterville, Maine, was among those who supplemented medical practice with other activities. He operated a distillery to make whisky from potatoes, conducted religious services and sold real estate.

In 1866 Lewis Pilcher graduated from the University of Michigan and opened a medical practice in Flint. He made many friends, but acquired no patients. He moved to a small settlement nine miles away where he gained an occasional patient. When there was no teacher available for the local school, he offered himself and became the village teacher and doctor. "I was making a living," he wrote.

Through the 1800s many Midwestern doctors farmed simultaneously. Some farmed all day and made their medical calls at night. They commonly gave up medicine to give full attention to their farms.

Some doctors ran drugstores for auxiliary income. One practiced medicine and sold coffins. It was common for the doctor to also be the postmaster and not unusual for him to double as the sheriff.

There was a revival of the earlier colonial practice wherein the doctor was also the preacher.

The story of a Kansas woman of this period tells how her doctor had married her parents, presided over her birth, christened her in church, performed her marriage ceremony, treated her in her last illness, and preached her funeral sermon.

In Wisconsin a doctor who was also a minister, druggist, and undertaker advertised, "I can handle you from the basket to the casket."

A versatile doctor in Kentucky sent the following bill to the executor of an estate:

Seventeen visits $8.50
Shaving the corpse $0.10
Preaching the funeral service $1.50
   TOTAL $10.10

When the great rush to California took place in 1849, it is estimated that as many as fifteen hundred medical men rushed along to the Golden State. Of course, most of these "medical men" did not have degrees. The Civil War made things worse. In Wichita, the largest city in Kansas, most of the doctors did not have degrees. Most of them were "Civil War veterans with a hankering for medicine." The story of one such doctor illustrates the way this came about.

He was a farmer who left his farm to fight in the Union Army. He was used first as a nurse, then as a cook, and late in the war he was detailed to dispense drugs. When the war ended he returned home and practiced medicine.

The difficulty making a living as a physician lasted a long time. In 1896 a Colorado medical journal reported that "seventy-eight physicians are licensed to wait and starve in Colorado while a practice is forthcoming."

Some medical journals offered advice on building a practice: "Wash your hands before examining a patient, not afterward" and "A useful attribute for a doctor is a good memory for names." One doctor told that he knew the names of every child, every dog and most of the cats within a ten-mile radius of his home. A journal cautioned to be careful "not to ask an unmarried woman how many children she has had, not to speak of a man's wife as his mother or of a woman's husband as her father, or worse of a lady as a man's wife when she is not." And another journal pointed out that "the very smile that makes 80 of your patients like you, is the very thing that estranges another 10."

There were a few irregular activities that might sustain a doctor who was waiting for patients and attending the girls of the local brothel was one. In San Antonio in 1910 the payment for a medical call at the brothel was five dollars. That was generous. House calls in San Antonio brought only two dollars.

And there were some memorable satisfactions to be derived from work in a brothel. Dr. Ferdinand Herff told how the mistress of a San Antonio brothel became pregnant in the course of an exclusive arrangement with a wealthy client. All of the girls became interested in the forthcoming event and contributed caps and coverlets. The doctor wrote that: "No birth was ever more happily anticipated." And he added that when it took place, the effect was more telling than the most fiery exhortation of the most fervid evangelist. One pretty inmate burst into tears when she saw the baby, checked out, went home, and married a friendly farmhand.

There was one very special aspect of waiting: The doctor

was also waiting to get married. That is, usually. In 1828 Dr. Samuel Gross had no patients and no money after his first-year in practice in Philadelphia. But he married anyway. "Of course we were foolish," he wrote, "very foolish, but how could we help it?"

A Texan set down a definite reference for the girl he planned to marry. Pat Nixon graduated from Johns Hopkins in 1909. He told his sweetheart that they would marry as soon as he was making one hundred dollars a month. In his first month of practice in San Antonio he collected fifty-seven dollars and the prospect for marriage seemed dim. But it took only four months to achieve the goal — and the girl.

A multitude of problems can complicate a doctor's plans for marriage. An emergency might disrupt the wedding day; it might even disrupt the marriage. In 1905 Dr. Asa Collins had his practice established in northern California. He was ready to leave town with the girl who would be his bride; they would travel to Sacramento to be married. There was one call to be made before they left.

To his dismay Dr. Collins found a twelve-year-old girl in labor, deserted by her boy friend and living with a blind grandmother. He delivered the baby, and to cover the affair — at the mother's urging — he took the baby.

With the baby in his buggy he proceeded to pick up his fiancee who came rushing out to meet him, bags in hand, and hopped into the carriage. She "stiffened" when she heard a feeble wail. "What's that?"

And when she found out, she said: "Stop. Take it back. I won't have it. What will people think?"

Then she picked up the baby and after a moment she was caressing and cuddling it.

As they drove on, Dr. Collins began to worry about this arousal of maternal instincts. If this went on for long he risked becoming a foster father before he was married. He stopped at a county hospital and gave the baby to a doctor friend for disposition. As they drove off from the hospital. Dr. Collins and his fiancee argued. She was concerned — poor child — let's go back and get it! She was in tears and he was in a huff on their way to their wedding.

Dr. Benjamin Gordon practiced in Philadelphia in 1900. He had a flourishing practice, he was thirty, he was open to marriage, and he was Jewish. These attributes made him the special concern of a remarkable institution: the marriage brokers.

The marriage brokers, for a fee, found husbands for marriageable Jewish girls. Dr. Gordon was besieged with offers: "Jews with long beards and skull caps... and women busy-bodies... infested my office and haunted my reception room. Rabbis from Worcester, Massachusetts, and Wilmington, Delaware, visited me with various wonderful and allegedly altruistic matrimonial propositions." They even posed as patients to get access to the doctor. It ended only when the doctor married a girl not listed on the brokers' rosters.

One doctor advertised, in a magazine, for a housekeeper. The ad stated that the job could lead to marriage. With that known to both parties, it was not surprising that it did.

There is a well-known downside to marrying a doctor. Dr. C.W. Mayo stated it: "I'd never advise any girl to marry a doctor. She will be in for a lot of loneliness." Today, when it is common for medical students to marry, a woman's hopes may crash in stages. She understands that there is little time for companionship in the face of the demands to be met in medical school; she hopes that it will be better after graduation. But being married to a resident is worse — and this lasts for several more years. She hopes that it will be better when he begins to practice — but it only gets worse.

A surgeon tacitly acknowledged his detachment when he queried his wife about their second child. He didn't remember their first child crying so much — getting him up so often at night. His wife reminded him that when their first child was born he was on hospital duty and was never home at night.

An obstetrician related what it was like to be married to a specialist in his field when he described his wife as "a self-sufficient entity who sleeps in the equivalent of a firehouse without resentment."

One doctor's wife saw a positive side to the demands made on medical marriages and called it to the attention of newcomers to her circle: "You needn't worry about tiring of each other," she said. "You won't spend enough time together."

But Louella May Berry saw unlimited opportunity for gratification and accomplishment in a medical marriage. In 1906 Dr. Fred Albee, a young orthopedist in New York, took Louella to concerts, on ferry rides, and on outings to Coney Island. The possibility of marriage began to take some form in their minds and Louella wrote: "After being associated with this fellow for a while, I realized that he was a genius and needed someone to work with him and help him.... Here was a golden opportunity for me to aid this young doctor to make a success of his life — and thus help humanity as a whole."

Her husband's public speaking needed to be improved. When he spoke at a medical gathering, Louella went along.. "I would take a seat in the back of the room. If I could not hear him, I would stand up and as soon as I could hear again, I would sit down." Dr. Albee, Louella May, and humanity were all being served.

But Louella May Berrys are in short supply — how to find a suitable mate? Dr. William Osier of Johns Hopkins, a source of wisdom on all medical subjects, included advice on marriage in his pronouncements to his followers: "Choose a freckle-faced girl for a wife," he said. "They are invariably more amiable."

He never revealed the basis for this prescription, but his authority is considerable and to date no studies have contradicted it.

Some marriages are inspirationally conceived. Dr. Warren

Cole waited long and patiently for his inspiration. At the age of forty-three, well into a distinguished surgical career, he was appointed professor of surgery at the University of Illinois School of Medicine. He came to Chicago from St. Louis and sought an apartment. As he walked in the hallway of a building with an available apartment, "I got the shock of my life. Walking towards me was a young woman. I glanced at her to see if I knew her, then stopped in my tracks, I glanced at her a second time. Yes, there could be no question about it — she was the girl I was going to marry..." He sought her acquaintance and married her.

In Boston, surgeon Claude Welch was similarly inspired. He first saw his future wife, a nurse, hurrying down a corridor at the Massachusetts General Hospital and knew at the moment that she was the woman for him. But just what inspired him remains a mystery: "Queerly enough," he wrote, "I cannot recall whether she was walking toward me or away from me."

8.

Distaff Doctors

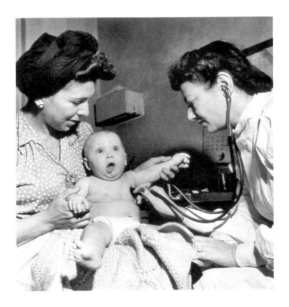

From the time of the ancient Greeks, the followers of Asclepius comprised a fraternity. American individualism and disdain for tradition was bound to challenge this heritage. The challenge came in 1846 when Elizabeth Blackwell, a young music teacher in Charleston, South Carolina, decided that she would become a doctor.

Miss Blackwell consulted several physicians in Philadelphia for advice: How should she proceed?

One doctor laughed at the thought of it; the idea of a young woman wishing to be a doctor was preposterous, Another suggested that she go to Paris. She would be allowed to attend medical school lectures there though she could not gain a degree. It was a futile suggestion. Elizabeth Blackwell wanted a medical education and she wanted one crowned with a degree. A third doctor suggested that she disguise herself as a male to gain admission to an American medical school and even offered to help her pull it off. Most of the doctors she visited advised her to give up the idea.

Elizabeth applied for admission to the four medical colleges in Philadelphia and to others in New York. All applications were rejected. Then she applied to twelve smaller medical schools and was rejected by all of them — except one. The faculty of the Geneva Medical College, in western New York State, asked the student body of the college to vote on the issue of admitting a female student. The students voted unanimously to admit Elizabeth Blackwell. The year was 1847.

The student vote was a magnificent, enlightened gesture. But it was said later that the students thought that the application was a hoax perpetrated by a rival medical college, and that they voted for admission to go along with the joke — that they were surprised when Miss Blackwell really showed up.

On arrival she was the object of much scrutiny by the community of Geneva. The women of the town stopped and stared at her when they passed her in the street — as though she was some curious animal, Miss Blackwell said. The community consensus was that either she was a bad woman or insane, and that one or the other of these qualities would manifest itself shortly.

But Elizabeth Blackwell was a diligent student with a winning personality. She was individually applauded when she graduated and most of the women of Geneva, as well as many from the surrounding territory, came to witness the event and join in the applause.

Her graduation was noted in London: *Punch,* the British humor sheet called attention to it and chided English women in a verse:

Young ladies all, of every clime
Especially of Britain
Who wholly occupy your time
In novels or in knitting
Whose highest skill is but to play,
Sing, dance, or French to clack well
Reflect on the example, pray
Of excellent Miss Blackwell.

Why would a young woman want to be a doctor? When Elizabeth Blackwell was twenty-four and teaching school, a career in medicine had been suggested to her by a friend. She rejected the idea: "I hated everything connected with the body and could not bear the sight of a medical book." She was an attractive girl and often lovestruck by boys, but "whenever I became sufficiently intimate with any individual to be able to realize what a life association might mean, I shrank from the prospect." Medicine offered her an intellectual challenge and independence.

Other young women had the same motives that led young men to study medicine, and one additional one — the fact that there was a barrier made some want to breach it. Anne Walter Fearn, who subsequently spent forty years in China as a medical missionary, grew up in Mississippi. Women doctors were tabooed in the South. "It was a question of propriety as to whether or not they should even be discussed in polite society."

Anne Walter decided to study medicine in 1889 and wrote to her mother. Her mother replied by wire: "No disgrace has yet fallen on your father's name. Should you persist in carrying out your mad determination to study medicine, I shall never again recognize you as my daughter."

And Dr. Anne Walter Fearn recalled: "That settled it. I just had to study medicine."

Josephine Baker considered medicine as a career in 1894.

When she mentioned it to her family physician he became "sulfuric." Her mother was "overwhelmed" and both sides of the family were "aghast." "When I encountered only argument and disapproval, my native stubbornness made me decide to study medicine at all costs and in spite of everyone."

Eliza Mosher was a member of the first class to include women at the University of Michigan in 1871. Her mother opposed her career choice. She said, "I would just as soon think of paying to have you shut up in a lunatic asylum."

Fathers were even less likely to approve, and they had the mothers to consider. When Bertha Van Hoosen sought a medical education at the University of Michigan in 1885, her mother cried every time the subject was mentioned. Her father said that he would surely not give financial support to anything that kept her mother continuously upset.

Medical figures were equally unsympathetic. Even that humanist Dr. William Osier at Johns Hopkins was vigorously opposed. When Dorothy Reed came to Baltimore for a pre-admission interview in 1900, she took a streetcar to the medical school and found herself seated opposite a man who studied her from head to foot and so continuously that she was discountenanced by it. He got off the car behind her and soon overtook her on the walk. He asked, "Are you entering the medical school?" Miss Reed gasped a "Yes," and he said, "Don't. Go home," and walked ahead of her into the hospital. It was Dr. Osier.

As more girls entered medicine, parental and professional objections diminished and motivations multiplied. Nancy Andreason was an author/English professor when she suddenly decided to remake her life (1966) and become a physician.: "I had my first child and finished my first book at about the same time.

"In thinking about the delivery, which had been complicated, I compared it to the work involved in the writing of my book. When I realized what even one physician accomplished in one childbirth, I admitted its superior importance over anything I could do as an English professor and decided to change my life."

Joni Magee elected medicine because the prospect for marriage seemed dim: "There wasn't anyone around to marry, I think if someone respectable had asked me to marry him, I probably would have and given up the idea of becoming a doctor. I couldn't catch a Jewish doctor, so I had to be one."

And to deal with the most erroneous of supposed motivations for the study of medicine, the advice given to a young woman approaching a pre-admission interview is indubitably correct. It came from a college professor who was her counselor. He warned her not to say that she wanted to help suffering humanity. She would be regarded as either a fool or a liar.

With Elizabeth Blackwell's graduation, a social barrier had been breached, but dissidents rushed to the barricade. When Elizabeth's sister Emily applied for admission to the medical school at Geneva, she was rejected. Nor was any other woman ever allowed to follow Elizabeth Blackwell at the Geneva Medical College.

Emily was accepted as a student by the Rush Medical College in Chicago, but the college was promptly censured by the Illinois State Medical Society and she was forced to withdraw. She was fortunate to find a place at the Western Reserve Medical College in Cleveland and she graduated in 1854.

At that time there were four female students among a couple hundred men at the Cleveland college.

The women had a box seat to themselves in the teaching amphitheater where they were "unmolested by the tobacco-chewing and spitting." The men wanted them excluded completely. They circulated a petition demanding it, and the faculty compromised by agreeing not to admit any more women.

At Harvard, Harriet Hunt had applied for permission to attend the medical lectures in 1850. Her request was rejected. The Harvard medical students protested that "no woman of true delicacy would be willing in the presence of men to listen to the discussion" of medical subjects and that they objected to having the company of any female forced upon them "who is disposed to unsex herself and sacrifice her modesty." Harvard did not admit a female to its medical school until 1945.

It is clear that men opposed women entering the medical profession in a very great part because the men could not handle the adjustment of personal relationships that it required. It embarrassed them.

In 1865, when women students were first allowed to attend lectures at the Philadelphia Hospital (Blockley), eminent surgeon Hayes Agnew tried to drive them away by exhibiting a nude male patient and appealed successfully to the hospital board to bar them.

In the same city, Dr. Wier Mitchell, famous neurologist, psychiatrist and novelist, acknowledged that he could not bring himself to discuss medical subjects in front of women. And in Baltimore, when the Johns Hopkins Medical School came into being in 1893, Dr. William Welch, who was the guiding light, opposed admitting women because he would have trouble saying things in the classroom that women might regard as indelicate. When Johns Hopkins did admit women, persuaded by a gift of a half million dollars from a women's group, a distinguished pathologist, Professor William Councilman, resigned in protest.

Years later, a daughter of Dr. Councilman studied medicine in a coeducational medical school. And after it was forced upon him and he had experienced it, Dr. Welch recanted and approved the idea of women physicians.

The male medical students had greater difficulties accepting women than the professors did.

Anatomy, the basic first-year course, focused the conflicting concepts in the men's minds and required a sharp psychological adjustment. Elizabeth Blackwell described the emotional tumult caused by her presence at an anatomy demonstration: "A trying day... dissection was just as much as I could bear. Some of the students blushed; not one could keep in a smile and some who I am sure would not hurt my feelings for the world held down their faces and shook. My delicacy was certainly shocked... but I sat in grave indifference, though the effort made my heart palpitate."

The class disruption was such that Miss Blackwell was asked to absent herself from some anatomical demonstrations. She wrote a note to the professor. She said that she was a serious, reverent student of anatomy and she thought that requiring her absence was a mistake, but that she would comply if the class wished it. The professor read her note to the class. They applauded. Miss Blackwell resumed her seat and everyone, including the professor, seemed relieved. All concerned had made a critical adjustment.

This unease in the anatomy laboratory persisted for a long time. In 1902, Mary T. Martin studied medicine at the North Carolina Medical College. But she was not allowed to study anatomy. It was thought improper for her to be in a room "with all those naked cadavers."

Pauline Stitt studied medicine at the University of Michigan in 1929. She shared a cadaver for anatomical dissection with another female student and two male students. On the day that dissection of the male genitalia was the assigned subject, all of her partners reported sick. Miss Stitt dissected the male genitalia resolutely while the class watched to see how she handled the trial. "I may have need for this experience some day," she told herself, but, "it wasn't a pleasant afternoon."

As with the men, some women had personal difficulties with anatomy. Irma Gross began her study of anatomy at New York University. She entered the laboratory and almost immediately became nauseated and light-headed. She had to leave. She sat outside and prayed that her agitation would cease. She must not be sick. To become a doctor she must spend several months in this laboratory. She regained her composure and reentered the anatomy hall. She experienced several similar episodes, but she struggled through them and then they gradually ceased.

The widespread opposition to the admission of women to the nation's medical schools induced a reasonable solution. In 1850, the Quakers in Philadelphia established a medical school for women. There were several male physicians in the founding group. The school was called the Female Medical College of Pennsylvania — the first such medical college in the world.

New barriers were raised immediately by dissidents. The students at the Female Medical College were refused study privileges at all Philadelphia hospitals. Worse, the Philadelphia County Medical Society refused to admit women to membership and ruled that its members were prohibited from teaching in the women's college and even prohibited from consulting with a woman physician in any medical case.

It was not until 1868 that students from the Female Medical College were allowed to attend the teaching clinics at "Blockley," Philadelphia's hospital for the poor. As mentioned, they had been driven away when they tried to attend in 1856. In 1868, the women students tried again. The men bristled, the instructors made it as unpleasant as possible for the girls by their selection of cases and topics, and the male students filled the air with denigrating remarks.

But the women came early and sat resolutely in the front row seats. One day during a surgical demonstration, the supply of pre-threaded needles gave out and two interns with sticky blood on their hands were unable to thread a new needle for the surgeon. The surgeon waited impatiently and finally ordered the interns to pass the needle and thread to one of the women. The nearest one received it and "with a quick and dexterous movement," threaded the needle and passed it back. The surgeon smiled and the students put aside their animus and applauded.

This was not a breakthrough in Philadelphia. In the following year, 1869, students from the Female Medical College were allowed — by the hospital board — to attend clinics at the Pennsylvania Hospital, the hospital associated with the University of Pennsylvania, but they were not welcome. The male students jeered and whistled when they arrived, threw wads of paper and quids of tobacco at them when they were seated, and threw stones at them as they departed. Dr. Hayes Agnew, the professor of surgery, resigned rather than teach before a mixed group. He expected that his resignation would force the women out, but the hospital board stood firm.

Women were admitted to the medical schools very cautiously and in limited numbers. At admission interviews they were asked if they intended to get married, if they intended to get pregnant and even what contraceptive they were using. And very commonly they were asked the question that infuriated them most: Have you considered being a nurse instead? There was an unwritten female quota of five percent that prevailed across the land into the 1960s.

At first, when the girls found places in the schools there was much amusing gender segregation.

The University of Michigan admitted the first woman to its medical school in 1870. The school had a red line painted on the floor of the amphitheater, running from the pit to the topmost row, and confined women to one side of the line. The red line endured at Michigan until 1903.

In 1916, Louise Farnam earned a degree in physiological chemistry at Yale. She wanted to study medicine. Yale had never had a female medical student. Miss Farnam was told that there was an insurmountable barrier to her enrollment. There was no women's bathroom in the school. Her father offered to pay for the construction of a suitable lavatory and his offer was accepted. Then Louise Farnam and two other women were admitted to the medical school. Miss Farnam graduated in 1920. Subsequent female medical students at Yale dubbed their lone lavatory the Louise Farnam memorial.

Concessions to gender created some comical innovations as the curriculum diversified. At one large university in 1940, the 120 male students stripped to the waist and listened to each other's chests to learn how to use a stethoscope. The five women in the class were isolated in a nearby women's rest room where they listened to one another's lungs in front of the toilet stalls.

As the female students examined each other, employees drifted in and out of the rest room.

Occasionally a male instructor stuck his head through the door blushing a bit as he asked the young women how they were making out. In such intervals the employees in the toilet stalls sat patiently, declining to come out until the doctor left.

When instruction shifted to examinations pertinent in obstetrics and gynecology, the women had a definite advantage. The men learned how to do a pelvic examination on a rubber model while the secluded women examined each other. The men were insecure after this exercise, but the women were confident.

But to learn something about urology a woman had to be a sleuth. At the Medical College of Virginia in 1930 they were "excused" from attendance at the urology clinic. That meant barred. At the end of a series of lectures on the subject there was a lecture on sexual problems, but the women were excluded. At the University of Kansas, women just didn't take urology.

At New York University in the 1940s, Irma Gross was assigned to the urology clinic, but in this instance laymen's customs and habits frustrated the educational effort: "I reported to the clinic the first day, but when I saw three patients frantically reach for their trousers as I entered the room, I decided to stay away. That completed my urologic training for the third year."

Of course, even conscientious disavowals of intent did

not keep students from getting pregnant, and a series of new scenes appeared on the medical stage. Reactions by the schools varied. Inevitably, denial was one of them. In 1954, a married, pregnant student in one of our medical schools, in her senior year, was called to the dean's office and told that her pregnancy would embarrass both her classmates and the school at graduation ceremonies. She was told that she must take the last semester off and come back and graduate after she had had her baby.

The medical milieu created other problems for pregnant students. Morning sickness might occur and it might continue for several months. The scenes and odors in a hospital were likely to aggravate the nausea.

At Kansas University, Marjorie Sirridge was into her residency when her pregnancy reached near term and nausea became a problem. She handled it heroically. She was on her hospital's obstetrical service.

She repeatedly delivered a baby, ran out of the delivery room to throw up and ran back in to deliver another baby.

Pregnancy in the course of a medical education would seem to be a maximum physical and intellectual burden for a woman to handle successfully. But Dr. Doris Bartuska demonstrated that women have enormous untapped strength and spirit. Dr. Bartuska had six daughters. She had the first when she was a junior in medical school, the second during her first year of hospital residency, two more before she completed her hospital training, and a fifth during a postgraduate fellowship.

The male medical students usually avoid dating the female students. They date the nurses instead.

The female students confront a dilemma. If they affirm their femininity, they are likely to be accused by the men of using their wiles to get grades, and if they are "one of the boys," they are susceptible to being seen as hardened and unwomanly.

They sometimes feel that they are regarded as a neuter

gender. One who pondered the dilemma and did not want to
sacrifice her femininity to medicine said: "I didn't want to be
known as the Buster Brown haircut and Oxford shoe type."

She said that male classmates saw the girls as sisters, not
women:

"When I'd go out with some of the guys, 1 was one of
their buddies. They'd confide in me and say, 'Nadine, there's
just no nice women to date.' I'd be sitting there thinking,
'My God, I'm here!'"

In 1969, the Female Medical College of Pennsylvania,
then called the Women's Medical College of Pennsylvania,
admitted a few men to its classes. In view of the abuse this
institution had taken in its early years, one might expect that
the men would encounter at least some jovial harassment. But
when one of the women students was queried on this point,
she dismissed it lightly and said that the men were treated
well — each of them just "as if he was one of the girls."

Some deans had multiple fears of ways their female
students might reflect undesirable images on their schools.
When Nellie Mattie MacKnight was about to graduate from
a medical college in San Francisco, she was asked how she
wanted her name on her diploma. She wanted it exactly as it
had been all of her life Nellie Mattie MacKnight.

At a conference, her dean repeated this affirmed name
several times and then said: "Can't you find something more
appropriate?" He went on: "What would you think if we were
to graduate a Doctor Willie or a Doctor Tommy with the
class?" Miss MacKnight was suddenly "faced with the need
of re-christening myself. She had an Aunt Ellen, she recalled,
and Helen of Troy came to mind for no discernible reason.

"You may write Helen M. MacKnight," she said, and the
dean stopped pacing the floor. "That's better," he said. "And
see that it is Helen M. MacKnight on your shingle."

The appropriate shingle went up, but she was well known
where she practiced and was known as "Doctor Nellie."

When the newly graduated distaff doctors sought

residency positions in hospitals, for further education, they encountered another obstacle: Hospitals did not want them. In 1932, 86 percent of the hospitals approved for residency training declined to take women.

In 1900, Dr. Dorothy Reed and Dr. Florence Sabin won appointments as residents (interns) at the Johns Hopkins Hospital by virtue of their academic achievements. But the superintendent of the hospital did not want them. He tried to compromise. He would take one of the young women, but the hospital could not take both because then one would have to work on the black male ward. The women countered that they were both quite willing to work on the black male ward. The superintendent was furious, so focused on narrow notions of propriety that he accused these two talented young ladies of harboring prurient sexual inclinations if they would accept such terms.

Male colleagues could be equally puerile. Dr. Emily Barringer was the first women appointed to the staff of a city hospital in New York, the Gouverneur Hospital, in 1903. On her first night of duty, she found that she had been assigned to do all necessary bladder catheterization on the male surgical ward.

It was obviously a challenge. She did them, most of some thirty beds, skillfully and with no comments from the patients. The seven men who comprised the rest of the in-hospital staff had played a high card and lost.

Mary Bates, the first female resident at the Cook County Hospital in Chicago, was similarly hazed.

The male residents once carried her off to the gynecology ward as an "interesting case" and another time to the morgue where they locked her in. But there came a third time when they carried her off to the amphitheater for a dinner in her honor for being such a hard worker and such a good sport.

Some traditions had to be breached. Dr. Ann Brace was the first female surgical resident at the Massachusetts General Hospital in Boston. The men all wore white shirts with "dog collars." Ann decided, "By God, I'm going to wear a blouse." She did, and each morning her senior resident would ask, "Ann, where's your uniform?" She responded that it hadn't come in yet. He said, "You'd better check," and she said, "Okay, I'll check."

This went on for months and Ann decided that she was never going to wear the dog-collar shirts.

Then one morning the senior resident said, "Ann, that's a pretty blouse," and that was the end of it. Ann mused that he was married to a very nice woman and she probably had talked to him.

Women learned how to be recognized as equals. Dr. Ruth Kimmelstiel spelled it out in 1953: "I could simply be smarter, work harder and complain less, and thus be equal."

In the early days there was an additional requirement: Occasionally the women had to be tough.

Resident Josephine Baker was called to see a woman in labor in a tenement district of Boston. The room was filthy, roaches were everywhere, four stunted children huddled in a corner, a drunken husband lay on the floor and the woman in labor reclined on a heap of straw. The woman's back was one large, ugly, infected sore. Her husband had thrown a kettle of hot water over her a few days before.

Miss Baker's questions about the burn brought the husband to his feet threatening his wife and the doctor and lurching toward them. "I ran out into the hall," Miss Baker wrote. "He followed me as I had intended...he crossed the stair-head and... I doubled my fist and hit him. It was beautifully timed. I weighed hardly half as much as he did, but he was practically incapable of standing up... He toppled backward... and slid to the bottom of the stairs with a hideous crash. There was absolute silence... I went back into the room, pushed a piece of furniture against the closed door and delivered the baby undisturbed."

Residents (interns) rode in the ambulances when hospitals established emergency services in our large cities. Dr. Emily

Barringer was the first woman to draw this assignment in New York City at the Gouverneur Hospital in 1903. The city supplied a cap and uniform for male ambulance doctors, but there was no provision for a woman. Dr. Barringer was given equivalent funds and told to supply her own uniform.

She considered wearing bloomers, which many strong minded women advocated at that time, but she feared that bloomers might attract undesirable attention. She needed a skirt short enough to allow vigorous activity, but long enough to preserve modesty.

While she was contemplating a design, she received a letter from a women's tailoring firm in Boston offering to design a suitable uniform for the first female ambulance surgeon. They devised a divided skirt "with all the essential comfort and safety features of bloomers." And they supplied it gratis.

The New York ambulance drivers were marvelously helpful to the first woman ambulance doctor.

When the ambulance came upon an unconscious man on a street corner, an immediate decision was required and it could be difficult to make: Was he drunk or could this be a head injury, perhaps a skull fracture? The driver's experience gave him a goodly measure of diagnostic insight. Dr. Barringer told how they often whispered in her ear, "Take him to the hospital, Doc," or "He's alright, take him to the police station."

Occasionally the proper designation was the morgue, or it might become the morgue on the way to the hospital. It was necessary to be alert and to make the right decisions. If an ambulance doctor brought a "deader" to the hospital, he or she was bantered and joshed unmercifully by the house staff. Some hospitals had an unwritten law that in such circumstances the ambulance doctor must provide drinks for the entire staff— a keg of beer.

The title "Doctoress" or "Doctress" was widely applied to the women doctors when they appeared. Women physicians decidedly did not like it. They were doctors and they wanted full recognition of it — the title died. "Hen-medic" persisted among derogators.

The increment of women physicians was slow and hospitals were slow to adapt to their presence.

Even in the 1970s, hospitals might have only a single mixed-use sleeping room for the resident staff on night duty. One female resident worried that her presence was disturbing one of the males who always slept on top of the covers with all his clothes on. But she was assured by other residents that he slept that way even when he wasn't sharing with a woman.

And there was always a question of how much clothing to remove for sleep because sleep was usually a series of naps interrupted by calls to various parts of the hospital. There is a much retold story about a female resident who was roused out for an emergency cardiac resuscitation and was seen sitting astride the patient, pumping on his chest, with her breasts swinging in and out of her gown with every maneuver.

Some vexations seem likely to be eternal. Being mistaken for a nurse is one of them. A female resident related her experience in the emergency room. "I always introduced myself as Dr. Spiegel and two minutes later they'd be telling their kid, 'Now open your mouth so the nurse can see.' With some of them, no matter how many times you made it clear that you were the doctor, if you were a woman, that meant that you were the nurse."

An equally obdurate annoyance is that of being measured unfavorably against the men. Dr. Toni Martin reconciled herself to it: "I came to terms with the fact that patients would always make eye contact with the male next to me because he looked like a doctor even if he was the pharmacy student or the orderly."

In addition to such special vexations, the female residents suffered all of those that stressed the men.

Fatigue was unending. Dr. Mary Bennett trained in San Francisco and had only an occasional day off. On one such day she and her fiance took a picnic lunch to a secluded, wooded spot for an outing. Her fiance was partial to Wordsworth, and after lunch he read her some poems. Dr. Bennett had been up all night promptly fell asleep. She slept all afternoon. She wrote that she thought it was an appropriate introduction to life with a woman physician. Her fiance was not a physician, but he seems to have passed the test. They were married.

The trials of the hospital residency training do what they are supposed to do. They transform hesitant, dependent medical students into self-confident, capable, and assertive young doctors willing and able to confront any challenge. Dr. Martin told how she and a group of girlfriends held a farewell dinner in a restaurant when they finished their hospital training. Six self-assured, forthright young women, enjoying each other created an unusually winning scene. A semi-inebriate at the bar watched for some time, obviously impressed, and curious. Then he approached the table and asked, "Are you girls astronauts?"

When the first women doctors were ready to practice — when they opened their offices — their adversities soared. Elizabeth Blackwell chose to practice in New York City. She was barred from the established medical institutions in the city. She became the focus of insulting male remarks and actions, and the butt of denigrating anonymous letters. She wrote: "I understand now why this life has never been lived before... it is hard."

Maria Zakrzeska, who graduated from medical school in Cleveland in 1856, was repeatedly refused both lodging and office space when she sought them in New York. People suspected that she was a bad woman.

And the men continued to test them meanly. After graduating from the University of Michigan's medical school in 1880, Dr. Bethena Owens returned to Roseberg, Oregon, to practice. A few days after she arrived she was invited by male doctors in the community to attend an autopsy. When she arrived, she was told that the autopsy was directed primarily at the genitalia of the male being examined and then she was offered a knife and invited to do it — an old challenging gambit. When she accepted the test, the news spread rapidly and a crowd gathered to watch. When she finished, the crowd gave her three cheers. But the town's women were shocked and many men expressed disgust. There was even talk of tar and feathers.

Dr. Owens had to move to Portland and make another start.

Who would consult a woman doctor who opened an office in the nineteenth century? Dr. Eliza Mosher opened hers in Poughkeepsie in 1875. She was surprised by the "assurance with which women came to my office and asked for illegal operations. That is what they thought women doctors were for."

Some came by mistake. Dr. Bessie Efher opened a practice in a small Iowa farm town. Her shingle read Dr. B.L. Efher. Her patient wanted a doctor for his wife and it generated this exchange; "I am the doctor." "Well, I'm looking for a real doctor, like other doctors," "I'm a real doctor like other doctors."

"Is there no other doctor in town?" "None." "Very well then, come, she cannot wait much longer."

And the women were used. Dr. Mary Dole opened a practice in Greenfield, Massachusetts, in 1891 and told about a man who came for her on a stormy night. He wanted her to see his daughter. He said, "When the night is so bad that the men won't go, we know we can get you."

Some came expecting a bargain. Dr. Alfreda Withington practiced in Pittsfield, Massachusetts, beginning in the 1890s. She told of an early patient who was taken aback when she presented her bill for services. "Why," he said, "I might have had a man doctor for that!"

The paucity of patients willing to consult female doctors made beginning practice very difficult. In Baltimore, Dr. Lillian Welsh joined with another woman doctor to open an office. Getting started was a mix anxiety and anguish: "The proverbial wolf howled loudly at our door, patients were few and far between, and our office hours were periods of solitary confinement."

And in New York City, Dr. Josephine Baker took in $185 during her first year of practice. She was once down to her last two dollars which, "I defiantly spent on a grand lunch at the Waldorf Hotel and a magazine to read on the trolley car going home." When she reached her office-apartment, a patient was waiting, "who paid me in cash and enabled me to carry on."

The female doctors also encountered occasional kindness, appreciation and consideration which reassured them that their undertaking was worthy of the toll. In Chicago in the 1890s, Dr. Bertha Van Hoosen had to rent a horse to cover the distance over which she made calls. When she rented a horse for several consecutive days, her stableman advised her to buy the horse. She didn't think she had enough money to buy a horse, she said, and the stableman asked how much she could pay. Bertha thought she could spend seventy-five dollars. It was insufficient, but the stableman said, "You may have the horse and I will throw in the harness, buggy, lap-robe, and a whip." And shortly thereafter, a patient told her that she needed a dog to watch the buggy and horse — and gave her one.

9.

Charging Too Much

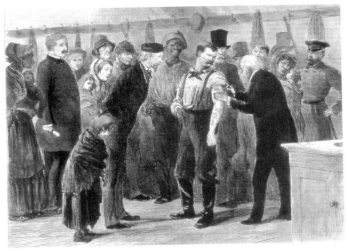

Vaccinating the poor

D octors have always charged too much; they have charged too much and not given sufficient time to their patients. And this will always be so because:

> Should he call upon his patients every day when they are ill,
> His motive plainly is, to make a great big doctor's bill.
> If he visits them less frequently — thus less'ning their expense,
> The chances are he'll be accused of wilful negligence.

Nonetheless, solutions date from 1643 at the Massachusetts Bay Colony. At that time Governor John Winthrop considered a proposal that healers in the colony not be allowed to ask any recompense. The doctor should be satisfied to receive "what God shall put into the head of the partie to give him."

Our colonists were high minded, but not so visionary as to generally embrace this solution. At the nearby New Haven Colony, the governor, who was also a busy healer, thought that some recompense was reasonable. In 1658, he asserted that not paying the doctor was "an act of unrighteousness," and that those who were at fault should pay up and not discourage the doctors.

Even the clergymen-healers of colonial times were not disposed to let the Almighty set their fees.

The Rev. Dr. Gershom Bulkeley, the healer who dominated Connecticut medicine in the late 1600s and early 1700s, complained that "no body of men I venture to assert, loose so large a percentage of their business by the unwillingness of debtors..."

Thus the American stage was set for a continuation of the centuries-long farce in which the doctors charge too much and the patients refuse to pay.

Government offered a solution in 1736. The Virginia Assembly, in response to complaints that doctors were charging too much, passed an Act to Regulate Fees For Medical Practitioners. For a visit and prescription in town or within five miles of town, the doctor was allowed five shillings (a bushel of wheat sold for five shillings, a pound of tea cost ten shillings). For every mile over five the doctor was allowed an additional shilling and he was entitled to an additional allowance for each river crossing that he had to make on the call.

Virginia colonists added a few unofficial features to this schedule to be sure that they were not overcharged. They often bargained a fee before they were treated and the bargain often stipulated that if a cure was not forthcoming, no fee would be paid: the doctor might travel twenty miles, but if the patient died before he got there, if the baby was born, if the fever subsided, or if the abscess ruptured, the doctor deserved no payment.

But such stringencies had onerous consequences. Physicians had trouble making a living. In 1799, physicians in Baltimore announced that they were not charging too much; they were not charging enough.

They gathered together and set a table of fees that would be " in accordance with the high price of necessaries of life." And they reminded the public that they treated the poor gratis.

In 1821, the doctors of Nashville, Tennessee, also published a fee schedule in the interest of public tranquility. The fees were modest — one dollar for a house call in town and two dollars for a night call. There was an amusing supplemental charge for some night calls. If the call came to the doctor "after abed," the fee was five dollars. It was well to have a doctor who stayed up late.

But, surely, didn't doctors charge too much in subsequent years and grow fat at the expense of the unfortunate? The history is otherwise. Dr. Thomas Emmet, who became a renowned surgeon in New York City, told how he made calls in the tenement houses along the East River in 1850 for twenty-five cents a visit. And in 1862 a doctor in northwestern Pennsylvania told how he made calls on fifty patients during a smallpox epidemic and none of them paid him. While in Baltimore in 1890, Dr. John Finney, later a distinguished surgeon at the Johns Hopkins Hospital, found that a private patient who could pay anything was a rarity.

In 1897, house calls in Columbia, South Carolina, were two dollars and office visits one dollar, but Dr. William Weston recalled that "these fees were pronounced exorbitant by many and were seldom paid in full."

In Chicago in 1907, life was better. Dr. Paul Magnusen was beginning his practice; his average fee per patient was a dollar and a half. But there was the qualification that many of his patients could not pay. And in Philadelphia, a sterling surgeon wrote that in 1915 small fees or no fee was what he regularly received.

Dr. Arthur Hertzler, who opened his country practice in Kansas at the turn of the nineteenth century, described the burdens that doctors accepted. He was called to see a young woman said to have a high fever and to be in terrible pain. She lived in a neighboring town. The roads were rivers of mud requiring the doctor's team of horses to walk every step of the way — it took seven hours. When he arrived he was told that his patient was sleeping quietly and need not be disturbed. An abscess adjoining her private parts had ruptured, the fever had dropped and the pain had disappeared. It would doubtless now heal by itself. "Of course, having done nothing I was entitled to no pay. Five dollars for the team and fourteen hours on the road was all I was out."

Dr. Rush McNair was similarly abused. Practicing in Kalamazoo, Michigan, he was called out on a cold stormy night that caused him to lose his way and forced him to walk through an extensive marsh area leading his horse to the home of his patient.. When he arrived, he was told from a second-story window that he wasn't needed and warned not to make any charge.

Dr. Benjamin Rush advised young doctors how to avoid disputes about fees. He said: "Receive as much pay as possible in goods or the produce of the country. Men have not half the attachment to these things that they have to money."

In the early 1800s, doctors commonly advertised that they would accept payment in produce such as cheese, lard, tobacco, maple sugar, beef or whisky. In Ohio, a pair of leather shoes paid for a baby's delivery.

In Texas in the 1820-30 period doctors were often paid in cattle or hogs. Quilts, bedspreads, hams and canned fruits and vegetables were bartered for medical care in North Carolina in 1912. And in the 1930s, when times were difficult, a busy practitioner in Arkansas was receiving 30 percent of his income in bartered produce. Occasionally the bartering caused troublesome commodity congestion. One doctor mused, "How many Hubbard squash can I use in a day?"

Barter fostered unlimited innovation. Dr. Ferdinand Herff, who arrived in Texas in 1847, told how shortly thereafter an Indian he treated promised to bring him a squaw when he noticed that Dr. Herff did not have one. Three months later the Indian reappeared with a teen-aged Mexican girl to fulfill his promise. Dr. Herff declined, but a German immigrant in the same settlement did marry the girl.

A doctor might fare better with barter than he would have in a cash transaction. In Chicago during the 1920s, surgeon Joseph Jerger removed a diseased appendix from the daughter of a butcher. The butcher had very limited resources, so when the fee was discussed the doctor offered a proposition: a steak for his family once every two weeks for ten years in exchange for the surgery. On first thought, it seeemed a dubious proposal. The butcher wanted to think it over. He made his calculations overnight, and in the morning it was done.

Ten years seems like a very long time, but barter is leveling in the long run. In Philadelphia, young Dr. Chevalier Jackson dreamed of a new medical specialty, one that would deal exclusively with diseases of the throat and lungs and develop new methods of treatment. He wanted to tour the medical clinics of Europe for ideas and information, but he had no funds for it. A patient learned of his wish and offered an exchange: fifty dollars toward the cost of the European tour in return for the care of his larynx for the rest of his life. Dr. Jackson accepted.

Bartering was complicated by the difficulty that laymen were unlikely to value a doctor's services very highly. Surgeon Hugh Young of the Johns Hopkins Hospital staff vacationed at Cape May in 1904.

There were no garages in Cape May, so the doctor persuaded a man who ran a bicycle shop to shelter his car for a month for ten dollars.

In the course of the month, Dr. Young used a dollar's worth of oil from the shop and on one occasion the owner assisted with the repair of a punctured tire. Dr. Young noticed that the shop owner's daughter had a tumor of dilated blood vessels on her upper lip and told the father that he would be glad to remove it. The shop owner was delighted. He had been told that he would have to take his daughter to Philadelphia for surgery. He was pleased to save the expense of the trip and elated when Dr. Young said he would do it free.

Dr. Young persuaded two physician friends to help him, one to give the anesthetic and the other to assist. The supplies cost about five dollars: ether, antiseptics, and sutures. The operation took about an hour and the girl's lip healed perfectly without the slightest sign of deformity.

When Dr. Young was ready to return to Baltimore at the end of the month, he spoke to the owner of the bicycle shop to settle his account. The summing up was a surprise. The man said: "I've got it all worked out — ten dollars for the storage of your automobile, one dollar for oil, and twenty-five cents for helping you repair that punctured tire — but you've been very good operating on my child, so just give me eleven dollars and I'll call it square."

But barter endured. Dr. May Wharton practiced in the hills of Tennessee during the 1940s. After a round of house calls one day she arrived home with her pay: three buckets of blackberries, canned beans in jars, eight eggs and a couple of live hens.

Ordinarily the clergy are treated gratis. But a prominent Washington surgeon thought that this courtesy was not diminished by requesting some courtesy in return. When a Virginia clergyman required surgery, the surgeon proposed an exchange: no charge for the surgery if the minister would preach the surgeon's funeral service gratis — it was agreed.

There was an odd uncharitable practice that was widespread in colonial times and lasted well into the nineteenth century. Strangers were charged more than local residents and this was generally regarded as quite just.

A physician with a sense of humor might find recompense for his services in nonmaterial ways. A Vermont surgeon recalled his visits to see an impoverished Irish woman who lived in two rooms, one of which was a closet without light or ventilation. She suffered from bronchitis and was pale and weak. She needed fresh air and sunlight, but she was in bed most of the time — in the closet. The doctor suggested that she move her bed into the larger room — near the window. When she said she hadn't the strength, he suggested that perhaps some friends would do it for her.

When the doctor returned in a few days, she had not moved. She promised that she would solicit friends. But after three visits, she still had not moved and the doctor reiterated his suggestion more forcefully. "Docthor darling," said she, "what nade have I of the sun when yerselfis afther showin' me yer own blessed face every day of me life."

She could not pay a cent, the doctor wrote, and if she had, it would have been expended and forgotten. But he was paid with a bit of blarney, he said, that has "kept her in my memory for half a century with renewed pleasure every time I recall it. It was very good pay."

Another surgeon mused that the squeeze of a patient's hand can be very good compensation.

But character and benevolence do not pay bills. Some compromise is better. Patients at the Mayo Clinic often inquire about fees; the prestige of the clinic makes them apprehensive. Dr. Charles W. Mayo was always ready to allay apprehension — to an appropriate degree. He told patients, "This clinic wouldn't be thriving if the fees were exorbitant, so you can be sure that the fee won't be too high... and we have a special arrangement... if the fee seems too low, you have the privilege of adding to it." He was never troubled to explain the special arrangement. Inevitably there was one instance in which the fee was too low. A wealthy man was charged ten thousand dollars for an operation performed on his wife by Dr. William Mayo. When the charge came to Dr. Mayo's attention he sent four thousand dollars back along with an apology. It was a mistake, he said, an overcharge by the business office. The recipient returned the check and said, gallantly, that his wife was worth the full ten thousand.

And there are fees that warrant reconsideration — by all concerned. In San Antonio, Dr. Ferdinand Herff was consulted by the family of a boy whose limbs were paralyzed, and the cause was unknown. The boy had been seen by physicians in New Orleans who could not offer either a diagnosis or a treatment — they didn't know. Dr. Herff thought that the condition was untreatable. But he had just received a faradic battery electric stimulating machine from Paris; great medical things were claimed for it. So he tried it.

Within ten days the boy showed improvement, and in two months he was well. Dr. Herff declined any fee. He said it was an experiment and he did not understand it. The family forced five hundred dollars on him — a magnificent fee in those days (1890).

Dr. Herff was intrigued. He took the apparatus apart and found that there was no battery in it.

Dismayed, he returned the five hundred dollars, and said that he had been victimized and made a charlatan unknowingly. The boy's father wrote back, returning the five hundred dollars and enclosing an additional check for one thousand dollars, "because you are the most honest man God Almighty ever created." Besides, he added, "You cured my boy."

Persons who fear being charged too much devise some droll maneuvers to avoid it. A Kentucky doctor was surprised when a notably penurious man whom he had never before attended telephoned and asked that the doctor make a house call. The caller had studied his choice and to assure the success of his act, he rehearsed the doctor on the performance he expected. He said, "Even if you do charge more, it is usually just as cheap in the long run because you don't make so many visits."

Frugal patients weighed the difference between the cost of a house call and an office visit when they thought one or the other was necessary. Dr. William Macartney, who practiced in upstate New York, had an elderly patient who was frugal and "gruff as a grizzly," but basically good-natured. On one occasion the doctor set off to make a house call and encountered his patient on his way to the doctor's office. The old man brandished his cane and shouted, "Go back! Go back, damn you! Go back and make it half price."

A common ploy was to ask the doctor if he charged for questions; sometimes the desired information could be elicited free. Alert doctors smiled and answered, "Not at all, but I do charge for answers."

Occasionally a perfect opportunity arises for a doctor to remind a delinquent patient of his negligence. A doctor delivering a baby at home was asked by an anxious father if the baby was "marked." He was anxious about birthmarks. He owed the doctor a large amount for services long past, and the doctor replied, "Yes. It's marked C.O.D." It was a great riposte, but it did arouse some anger.

In small communities it was often widely known that some doctors made no efforts to collect overdue bills. Dr. Josephine Evarts, who began practice in Cornwall, Connecticut, in 1929, was one of these and she explained how it came about. She quickly accumulated a large backlog of unpaid bills and finally decided that it was time to go around and collect some of them. She repeatedly found herself in homes where there was no food in the refrigerator, and compassion drove her to the grocery store to buy a couple bags of food and allay the suffering. "After several years of doing that," she said, "I figured it was unprofitable to try to collect bills, I just let them go."

Occasionally a bill is paid long after it has been forgotten. A Michigan doctor told of a young man who came to his office and asked if the doctor had been paid for attending his birth. The doctor recalled that he had not, and the young man paid him immediately — with interest.

When charges are disputed it is common for patients to compare the disputed charge with a lower charge made by some other physician. Explanation is useless and argument is worse. The best counter is said to be, "I'm sure he knows the value of his services."

If a dispute is for a considerable sum, as for an operation or for intensive care over a long period, the doctor has an equally ultimate position: "It is still cheaper than the cheapest funeral."

Deadbeats, those who solicit compassion and then slink away, cannot be avoided. A sense of humor helps the doctor bear the insults. A whimsical verse tells of a doctor who, after death, is being escorted to his reward by an angel who murmurs, "Wait," and then:

> *I have a place to show you*
> *It's the hottest place in Hell*
> *Where the ones who never paid you*
> *In torment always dwell*
> *And behold the doctor saw there*
> *His old patients by the score*
> *And grabbing up a chair and fan*
> *He wished for nothing more*
>
> *Said the angel, 'Come on doctor*
> *There are pearly gates I see'*
> *But the doctor only murmured*
> *'This is heaven enough for me.'*

There is one recorded instance of a doctor attacking the deadbeat problem directly. In 1914 a young general practitioner was working hard in a small community, but he was not being paid. He noted that the grocery store was being run profitably, so was the theater and the liquor store. He was very busy, but he was not profiting — he was being abused.

He was called out on an ugly, foggy night and after a long drive found three drunken men and one woman in the after-stages of a party/fracas. There was blood everywhere; it came from a long scalp wound sustained by one of the men. The doctor shaved, cleaned and sutured the wound and when he was ready to leave, he asked the homeowner — the least intoxicated of the three men — for twenty-two dollars. The host looked surprised and said he would tell his friends when they sobered up in the morning.

The doctor lost his temper, "Now," he shouted. "You!"

The drunk enraged him further by saying, "You're crazy if you think I'm going to pay you."

The doctor wrote, "I have always been a very mild person," but he proceeded to knock the homeowner to the floor. When one of the other drunks rose from the floor, the doctor knocked him down and then knocked the first one down again as he rose from the floor. The doctor had the great advantage of being sober and angry.

When the men were under control, the doctor emptied the pockets of all of them onto a table. He helped himself from the funds available to a total of twenty-two dollars and left. When he recorded the event, he commented: "Needless to say I did not use this method of collecting a bill again."

But collecting one's due requires some aggressiveness. Dr. George Vandegrift, who practiced on the lower East Side of New York City in 1879, described a lesser variety of aggressive bill collecting. A patient who owed for three obstetrical deliveries and was making no effort to pay came to the doctor's office for a minor surgical procedure. The surgery was done under chloroform and while the patient was anesthetized the doctor and his assistant went through his pockets and found thirty-five dollars. They left two dollars and a receipt for past and present services amounting to thirty-three dollars. There was no complaint.

But who can read a heart and say "deadbeat"? When Dr.

Bertha Van Hoosen opened her practice in Chicago in 1892, she treated many women who were poor and could not pay. One woman who had paid for several visits appeared and said she had come reluctantly because she had no money. Dr. Van Hoosen treated her and said, "When you owe me I feel I have money in the bank. The important thing is to get you well."

The woman did get well, and she returned and asked if sixty dollars was the correct amount that she owed. Dr. Van Hoosen, not expecting to be paid, hadn't kept track of it —she had no idea — so she said, "That's correct." The patient paid and bid her an affectionate goodbye.

The next day the landlady of the apartment house reported that the woman had departed in the middle of the night — absconded. She owed three months rent, a gas bill, and most of the other tenants in the building.

And there are the poor. Doctors have always assumed special responsibility for the medical needs of the poor. But they recognize some categories within the designation. There are at least three. There are "God's Poor," those unfortunates who through no fault of their own are always in difficulty; the "Devil's Poor," those who live well and never pay if they can avoid it; and the "Poor Devils," those who were once reasonably prosperous and would gladly pay if they could. Doctors can be assured of at least one reward for treating all three groups: They will never be accused of charging too much. One doctor added another group, consisting primarily of the elderly disabled whom he never charged. He called them his "Kingdom of Heaven patients."

10.

The Pleasures
and the Pain

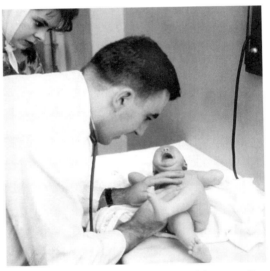

Doctoring is full of pleasures diluted by peculiar pains.
It is not for everyone; it has always been a rigorous
life. Theodorick Bland went to extraordinary lengths to
make himself a doctor only to find that he was unsuited for
it. Bland was born near Petersburg, Virginia, in 1740. As a
youth he traveled to England and Scotland for the best medical education available. He returned to Virginia in 1765 and
practiced medicine for seven years. Then he abandoned it:
"I have undergone all the distresses, cares and anxieties of a
conscientious practitioner of physic, and all this in direct opposition to my inclinations to a calm, quiet, and philosophical

life. My resolution to renounce the practice of physic is not the effect of whim or caprice, but of absolute necessity."

And doctoring requires equanimity. John Parks graduated from Dartmouth College and took up the practice of medicine in 1794. He ministered to the sick for some six years. Then he gave it up: "Pondering the miserable anxiety I have always felt when in charge of a patient dangerously ill, it seems to me that if I cannot conquer this useless sympathy, it will be most for my comfort to relinquish the profession and try some other method of supporting myself and my family." He started a newspaper.

And the doctor's equanimity must include a philosophical composure — doctors are not miracle workers. James Percival graduated from the Yale Medical School in 1815 and abandoned the practice of medicine after a very short experience. He said that he could not bear to have people look to him for relief and not be able to relieve them.

It is well when illusions of doctoring are tempered by reality earlier than they were in these men.

Dr. Ferdinand Herff told how an ambitious mother inspired her son inadvertently in the 1920s and directed him toward his proper destiny. The boy had decided to be a doctor and his mother asked to borrow some medical books from Dr. Herff. She hoped that the books would increase and fix her son's interest in medicine. Years later, the boy recalled how he opened a book to a color depiction of smallpox in its ugliest form — red, yellow and blue oozing pustules covering the entire body. He took one look, closed the book and decided instantly to study law.

Misconceptions of life as a doctor are almost the rule among young people seeking a medical education and they not infrequently misdirect a life. A woman physician after almost fifty years in medicine wondered: "How did I ever get into a life confined by renal tubules, cerumen and pus, when what I really like is art, music and social history."

For the novelist Walker Percy, a fortuitous event turned

a discontented doctor toward the path of his real bent. Percy was a first-year resident at the Bellevue Hospital in New York and increasingly dissatisfied with his lot. But he didn't know why and he had no plans to do anything about it. He contracted tuberculosis in the course of doing autopsies on patients dying from this disease and he was elated: "I was the happiest doctor who ever got tuberculosis. It was a great excuse to quit medicine."

A few individuals who find that they are marginally suited for the role they have chosen can mold themselves to meet the requirements and pursue a medical career with success and gratification. In the 1950s, Dr. Thomas Starzl completed an extensive surgical training program and was superbly qualified to fill any post with the most demanding surgical responsibilities. But, "the incongruity was that I did not like doing the one thing for which 1 had become uniquely qualified." He worried too much; apprehension related to surgical risks and responsibilities often made him sick. But he learned to worry less — even to dare. He became the pioneer and leader in the surgical field of organ transplantation.

Accepting a doctor's role may be difficult. The doctor learns quickly that one's best efforts, even his charity, will often be misconstrued, ignored, and even denounced. He has to accept it philosophically, and to a gradually increasing degree humorously — it is the human situation.

Colonial doctors faced notable physical demands as well as intellectual challenges. Outside of the cities, patients were widely dispersed. It was not uncommon for a doctor to travel fifty miles to see a patient. Before 1900 they usually rode horseback. In the winter they might make their calls on snowshoes. In colonial Connecticut, clerical healer Jared Eliot usually read a book as he rode horseback on his rounds.

When Eliot became engrossed in his book, his horse sometimes pursued an independent course and the doctor might rouse from his reading to find himself staring at an off the route haystack that his horse thought looked appetizing. In colonial times physicians were given a drink of rum wherever they called and they dined at whatever home they happened to be in at noon. One Connecticut doctor was said to enter the kitchen when noon was approaching, and to lift the kettle covers. If he liked what he saw, he stayed for dinner; if he didn't, he hurried on.

When eastern doctors had advanced to making their calls in buggies, the doctors in the Midwest were still in the horseback stage. In Indiana of the 1830s a doctor on horse-back might see forty to fifty patients on a round of twelve to thirty-six hours made over Indian trails, across rivers and ponds, and through great swamplands, covering fifty or sixty miles in the course of the circuit.

Dogs raced out from the houses along the route and often caused the horses to bolt. The doctors carried clubs to ward off the dogs; some carried a pocketful of stones to throw at the dogs. One doctor listened with interest when a farmer related an amazing tale of finding his dog dead with a stone stuck in its throat. The doctor had ridden past that farm with a pocketful stones on the very day.

At night in the Midwest, wolves were a threat. It was dangerous to travel alone. Doctors used the stars as guides during the night, and in storms they welcomed flashes of lightning that might reveal some familiar landmark. A doc-tor making a night call in Kansas told how his horse strayed off the road and carried him some way down the gulch of a dry riverbed before he recognized the error. And a doctor in Illinois was making his rural way on a night so dark he barely dared to proceed when he saw what appeared to be the wide portal of a covered bridge ahead. He directed his horse into it and found that he had passed through the open doors of a large barn creating a clamorous bedlam among the residing horses, cows, pigs and chickens.

Another doctor on a night call fell asleep in his carriage and his horses walked over a cow sleeping in the middle of the road. The doctor was awakened by what he thought was an earthquake with his carriage bouncing up and down violently as the cow tried to get up underneath the carriage.

In Kentucky of the 1870s a doctor wrote, "I rode yesterday 59 miles to see two patients, 32 to see one and 27 to see another." And a fellow Kentuckian related how after a day on his rounds with his horse he received a night call asking for help. He replied that his horse was too tired to go out again, but he would respond if the caller would come and get him. Some doctors kept two or more horses so that they would always be able to respond.

When railroads were established in the Midwest, doctors rode the rail cars when they could.

Engineers slowed the train so the doctor could drop off wherever he wished, rent a horse and proceed on his way. Scraped hands and bruised knees from dropping off the moving trains were common features of such trips. A Kentucky physician acquired a hand-propelled tricycle that fit the railroad track; he could stop at any point he wished, continue on, or return. If his timing was right he could put this tricycle aboard the train for the return trip. Inevitably he eventually met a train head-on while aboard his tricycle and jumped off just in time to save himself.

As the Midwestern farm states became more populated, a wire cutter, a wire stretcher, staples, and a hammer had to be added to the doctors' bags. It was often necessary to take a cross-country route to see a patient, and this might require cutting several wire fences on the way. The doctors usually repaired the fences.

But in winter snow drifts required detours off the trails into the fields, and back to the trail or road again, cutting a fence with each maneuver, and the maneuver might have to be repeated several times on a call. In the winter the doctors did not repair the fences; the farmers understood and were usually not resentful.

A Michigan doctor of the mid 1800s told how the farmers would came out of their houses as he passed by on a call.

They wanted some service or advice. Commonly they had a troublesome tooth, and the doctor extracted it at the roadside. The farmers hung a white sheet on the roadside gate if they wanted the doctor to come in. If the doctor encountered a complicated case, perhaps a difficult birth, he might stay four or five days at a home before he returned to his residence.

As roads were developed in the Midwest, doctors were able to use a chaise or a four-wheel carriage. Most doctors read as they traveled about, but some devised other recreations to pass the time. In Kansas, Dr. Hertzler entertained himself with a six-shooter. He shot at fence posts as his carriage jogged along. If a prairie dog, jackrabbit, or owl appeared, it made a more interesting target. He wrote: "I have fired as many as five hundred rounds on a single trip." For some doctors the pleasure of observing nature's beauties was ample reward for the tedium of long rural rides. Dr. Marcus Bossard was gratified by nature as he traveled about in southern Wisconsin in the late 1800s: "As the team followed a narrow wagon trail through the depths of the woods, I sometimes paused long enough to hear the call of the mourning dove or the whistle of the quail... and the plaintive song of the meadow lark often caused me to stop my team and listen... even saw the humor of a skunk walking leisurely and unconcernedly in the road ahead... as if he gloried in the advantage of his odorous weapon should danger approach too near... beautiful vistas among the wooded hills which changed with every turn... were recompense for the hardships of my profession."

Doctors' wives might accompany them on the long rides so they could spend some time together.

Carriages were easily upset on the rutted roads, and an assault by a dog was almost certain to lead to an accident. Dr. Hertzler described how the dogs lay in wait along the side of the road. They jumped at the noses of the horses causing them to swerve sharply and upset the carriage. Some dogs would jump at the side of a horse, grab a part of the harness in their teeth and hang on. The terrified horses raced forward and the doctor dared not shoot the dog — though it was legal to do so — for fear of hitting his horse.

Doctors learned what wonderful animals horses are. When the doctors fell asleep returning from calls, their reliable horses took them home. The horses knew when a stream was too deep to be forded, and they sensed when a bridge was under water or that part of it had been washed away, and they refused to proceed. Every country doctor told tales of being saved by his horses. They found the way home when the doctor was lost and they found the way in snowstorms in which the doctor would surely have perished except for his horses' sense of direction. Many nineteenth century doctors wrote more about their horses than they did about their patients.

The horses were less intuitive in their encounters with new inventions. In 1904, a Missouri doctor was returning home in a buggy at the end of a night consuming call and he fell asleep trusting his horses to take him home. The horses ventured onto a railroad crossing just as the train came along and both were killed. The carriage was destroyed, but the doctor, who was warmly dressed, was thrown free and escaped serious injury.

Some long calls turned into great comedies — in retrospect. In the 1890s Dr. John Wheeler, who practiced surgery in Burlington, Vermont, was summoned to see a young man on a farm some twenty miles away. He was told by the local doctor that an operation seemed to be necessary.

Accompanied by a nurse, Dr. Wheeler started off at 4 p.m. in a buggy pulled by two horses.

Shortly after dark, one horse stepped off the edge of a low bridge and fell into a brook. The carriage teetered and the doctor shouted for the nurse to jump. As she stood to do so, the horse lunged to its feet and threw her into the water. Then the horse started off with the carriage on its side and the doctor in the buggy top. Very shortly the carriage caught in a barbed wire fence with the doctor still in it and the horses ran off down the road.

A light gleamed nearby and Dr. Wheeler shouted for help. A farmer came and helped the doctor and the nurse gather their things and took them in. While the nurse dried out, the doctor went to look for the horses. He found that another farmer had captured them a short way down the road. The farmer repaired the buggy — it needed a new wheel — and then the surgeon and the nurse started off again on their call.

Arriving at his destination, Dr. Wheeler found a young man in a bad way due to intestinal obstruction. He operated immediately, on the kitchen table as it was done in those days, but the boy died.

His mother screamed, "You've killed my boy!"

The usual charge for such surgery was one hundred dollars, but the family circumstances seemed unpromising. Dr. Wheeler asked for fifty dollars and was given a check. The bill for the horses and the repair of the carriage was forty-five dollars and the doctor had ruined his raincoat when the carriage was dragged. The trip was neither a surgical nor a financial success, but Dr. Wheeler wrote: "It was an experience worth having even if it was decidedly less enjoyable when it happened than it is in retrospect."

Occasionally such calls were even pleasurable when they happened, as was one made by Dr. David Kellogg in Plattsburgh, New York, in the same era. "Last night I was called out to...They had a nice new baby and were happy. The night was very windy and the snow was flying. We tipped over three times, but were not hurt. My elbows were a little lamed. Got home about 3 a.m. I was so excited that I could not sleep. It was an experience."

But some experiences require a sterling sense of humor and the serenity of a saint. Dr. Robert Morris, a New York City surgeon of the early 1900s, told of a telegraphed request that he come to a city in the western part of the state and care for a woman with an ovarian tumor. She required an operation, the telegram stated, and a Dr. B., a physician known to Dr.

Morris, wished him to do it.

On arrival. Dr. Morris was met at the train station by a man with a farm wagon; there was no sign of Dr. B. The man with the wagon took Dr. Morris to a small house and said he would go for Dr. B. When Dr. B. arrived he seemed greatly surprised to see Dr. Morris; together they did the operation.

When Dr. B. took Dr. Morris to the train station he inquired how it was that Dr. Morris was called. When he was told of the telegram, he denied sending it and said the man "has not a dollar to pay you." For Dr. Morris, it was a twenty-four hour trip at his own expense and the loss of a full day in his office.

When Dr. B. asked the man why he did it, he replied, "Well you said the trouble was terrible bad and you wished that Dr. Morris was here, so I went and got his address and telegraphed him to come, because I wanted my wife to have the best there was." And Dr. Morris, with incomparable good humor, said, "It is worthwhile doing something for a man with that spirit."

On rural calls, after seeing a member of the household, doctors were commonly asked to look at a horse, or a cow, or even pigs. Laymen assumed that a doctor who could treat people would be equally capable of treating animals. Dr. Asa Collins attended a farm wife who was bleeding following childbirth and rescued her from a precarious situation by intense and prolonged effort. When she was safe and stable, her husband asked the doctor to follow him to the barn and led him to a cow with a calf half in and half out of her womb and stuck there. The doctor rigged up a block and tackle, roped the calf and gently the two men pulled it out safely.

As Dr. Collins left the farm the farmer paid him with two ten dollar gold pieces and said, "Thanks for saving the calf."

The conclusions suggested by that remark are confirmed by the report of a rural Texas doctor in 1841. He treated a young girl and prescribed for a sick sow. He charged two dollars for seeing the girl and three dollars for treating the sow.

And in Wyoming, Dr. William Hocker attended the wife of a rancher and saw her through a threatening illness. When it was clear that the woman would survive and the doctor took his leave, the rancher said, "Thank God you saved her, Doc. I'd rather lose the best critter on the ranch than Lizzie."

Many doctors of the late 1800s and the first quarter of the twentieth century were rough-hewn characters who brooked no nonsense from patients and had no time for hand-holding or what is now described as a bedside manner or TLC (tender, loving care). Their patient devotion was ardent, but it was also forthright. Patients recognized the integrity of these men and dealt with the gruffness sensibly.

A Midwestern orthopedist of the period was described as a man who smoked black cigars, blew smoke in his patients' eyes, roared at young mothers, and swore at the operating room staff as he threw surgical instruments on the floor. After he was dead, the community remembered him as a wonderfully kind man and named the local high school for him.

House calls created endless opportunities for comical misunderstandings. In the early 1900s, a Long Island doctor on a house call encountered a man with abdominal pain and recommended a soapsuds enema — two quarts of warm water well-sudsed with strong laundry soap. It is very effective. But "when I called next morning he received me coldly," the doctor wrote. The patient reported that he had done "nothin', but belch and puke up soap bubbles all night." The doctor was taken aback. "You didn't swallow it?" he asked. "What the hell do you think I done? Think I shoved it up my..." was the rejoinder. The doctor explained, but it was too late. He was dismissed. "I don't want no doctor what sticks medicine in my rear end. I takes my medicine through my mouth," the patient exclaimed.

The human behavior revealed on house calls is so diverse and so unique that it easily exceeds the most vivid imagination. The same physician told of calling at the home of a farmer whose wife was confined to bed because of weakness in her legs. As he approached the bedside, the farmer cautioned him:

"When you turn down them covers, Doc, look out for the aigs." The doctor turned down the covers carefully and found the bed full of chicken eggs placed closely around the lady's legs. The farmer said, "Mom can't do no housework... so I thought I'd put her to work hatching aigs."

There is a medical aphorism to the effect that probability is the rule under the skin. In medicine, certainty is dangerous and the patient's welfare is served when doctors are tentative. But some patients demand certainty and a doctor's tentativeness may provoke scorn. When a mother brought her teen-age daughter to a Texas doctor in the 1920s, the doctor examined the girl and said that he thought she was pregnant. The mother arose, threw two dollars on the doctor's desk and stomped out saying that she didn't want a doctor who "thinks," she wanted a doctor who "knows."

Another aphorism, "assume nothing," serves doctors better, but it is difficult to proceed without some assumptions. When an elderly gentleman complained of diminished vision, his doctor positioned him in front of an eye chart as is usual and directed him to read the top line of the chart: "Can you read that?"

The answer was "No."

"Can you read the line below?"

The answer was "No."

"The next one down?"

"No."

"The next line below, can you read that?"

"No, not a word," the man said. "I never learned to read."

New products and devices elicit novel reactions. A Michigan doctor laughed uproariously when he received a note from one of his patients requesting more medicine. He had given her quinine, a powder put up in capsules, for a recurrent fever. It was helpful she wrote, but she wanted it in some other form. She said that it was a great trouble to pick the shells off the medicine. Another said his patients referred to the capsules as "them thar tiny bottles," that he had to break to get the medicine out.

When medical clinics came into being, the pace of processing and the brevity of relationships created new situations for comedy. One busy doctor moving through examining rooms picked up the blank chart of a new patient, noting only that the last name of the patient was Poe. He entered the room and encountered an African-American teenager. The doctor introduced himself and in a friendly manner asked facetiously, "Are you any relation to Edgar Allen Poe?" The boys face lit up with a grand smile. "I is Edgar Allen Poe," he said.

When policemen, firemen, and new recruits for various services are being examined in groups at city clinics, some misidentifications are inevitable. Dr. Rosalie Morton examined recruits and members of the New York City Police Department at such a clinic in the early 1900s. The men were required to pass a yearly fitness examination. They were put through the tests in groups. The tests included hurdling barricades, carrying loads up and down ladders, lifting weights and wrestling with some skill. Near the end of one of the first series of tests a man dropped out of the group and declined to go on. "I came here to get a marriage license," he said, "I don't see that this is necessary." He was directed to another floor for his tests.

There are an infinite number of ways to misidentify a patient in a busy clinic. Dr. Richard Furman told of entering an examining room in a busy urology clinic and encountering an elderly man. The doctor plunged directly into the problem that usually brings elderly men to urology clinics: "You having some trouble passing your water?" The man stared at him in amazement, "Why yes, a little." Dr. Furman proceeded swiftly. "Do you have to strain to get started?" The answer was, "Yes, I sure do." The diagnosis was practically made. "Do you dribble when you finish?" The man grinned, "How did you know that? Amazing! You know all about me."

The doctor swept on to a few concluding statements, "I think we can help you with a relatively simple operation." Suddenly looking startled, the old man struggled to make a protest, "No, no," he said. "I don't need an operation, I just brung my wife in to see about some bladder trouble. She stepped out to the bathroom, but she'll be right back."

Contretemps such as that call for some quick thinking: the doctor must save face, he must maintain his dignity, and he must find a recovery position that maintains the patient's confidence. At the Mayo Clinic, Dr. Charles Mayo, one of the co-founders of the clinic, could do all of these things smoothly. On one occasion he was asked to see a woman who for one reason or another was dissatisfied with the opinions given by the Mayo staff. She had a multitude of complaints all of which were thought to be of nervous origin. She was unhappy with this diagnosis and therefore was directed to Dr. Mayo.

Dr. Mayo listened patiently as the lady poured forth every complaint known to physicians except faulty elimination. Dr. Mayo thought this was a clue to a way of resolving her dissatisfaction. When she finished he offered an authoritative opinion in an authoritative tone: "I think your trouble is constipation."

"But doctor," she countered, "I have a movement every day!"

Her response would seem to have destroyed Dr. Mayo's position. But he was unruffled; he remained authoritative and replied without a moment's hesitation or a flicker of uncertainty: "Yes, I know," he said, "but the trouble is that each movement is three days late."

Such mental agility has wide application. On one occasion when the Texas State Medical Association convened in San Antonio, the president rapped for order to open the meeting and announced: "Reverend Mr. Johnson will now pronounce the invocation." There was no response: no indication that the Reverend Mr. Johnson was present. "Is there a minister of the gospel in the house?" the president asked. Again there was no response, but the president paused for only a few seconds. Then he announced: "This session of the Texas State Medical Association will proceed having faith that the Lord will have mercy on us anyhow."

Even doctors of wide experience are regularly taken unawares by their patients and unexpectedly amused. Dr. John M. Warren had a very large practice in Boston during the mid 1800s. Among his patients was a poor woman whom he saw in his office over the course of many months. He never charged her because he knew she was impoverished. Then she ceased to come to his office. After an interval, Dr. Warren encountered her on the street and he asked politely why she had not been to see him recently. He meant to hold the way open for her, but her answer surely made —or unmade — his day. "I concluded to consult a pay doctor," she said.

Boston was also the site of similar contemporary drama of the unexpected — another comedy. A woman admitted to the Boston City Hospital was found to be at death's door due to neglected pernicious anemia. The hospital staff and visiting specialists worked heroically to save her life. The patient was so ill that she was barely aware of their efforts — all charitable of course.

She survived. The entire staff rejoiced in the triumph. They were proud of themselves and she was seen as their trophy. Their pleasure made her a celebrity in the hospital, until — almost as soon as she was able to do so — she requested that she be transferred to another hospital. She said, "I think the food would be better there."

The tragicomedies can scale great heights. In the 1930s, a Maryland farmer brought his son to the Johns Hopkins Hospital for examination. A medical review indicated that the "boy" was meant to be a girl.

The unfortunate child was born with malformed, mixed genitalia: she was a hermaphrodite. Fortunately, it appeared that a surgical solution could be effected without great difficulty.

When surgery was proposed, the child's father refused to consider it. The surgeon was astonished. Why would he refuse? The farmer was adamant. He explained that he already had six girls and besides, he needed this boy to work on the farm.

Does one laugh at the farmer's rusticity or ache over his ignorance and his offspring's misfortune?

It depends on one's mood, the occasion and one's company.

A similar tragicomedy unfolded when a ten-year-old girl with a disfiguring array of pimples on her face was brought to a hospital emergency room by her parents. They wanted the pimples treated.

The girl's appearance suggested masculinization which in turn suggested abnormal endocrine gland function. Skin changes due to the same process were the cause of her florid pimples. The doctors could feel a tumor deep in her abdomen, probably a tumor of the adrenal gland, the cause of the endocrine changes and an ultimately fatal affliction unless it could be removed. They urged that the girl be admitted to the hospital.

But the family balked. They were only interested in the pimples. When the father was told that the child had an endocrine disorder — that she was turning into a boy — he had a ready, simple solution. They would just change her name.

Some incidents arouse pure pain. There is a dark side to the human situation. Dr. Chevalier Jackson, practicing in Philadelphia, created new instruments and new techniques for removing foreign objects accidently lodged in the throat or lungs. His methods saved many children from death and were adapted to treat a variety of diseases. Early in his career a mother brought a small boy to the hospital. The boy had a quarter stuck in his throat. Dr. Jackson removed the coin and noted incidentally that the boy's body was covered with bruises.

The father came to the hospital to take the boy home and on leaving demanded that the quarter be returned. He was told that all such objects were being put into an educational collection display that would teach and demonstrate what sort of objects created dangerous medical problems in children and how the problems could be treated. Though the child had been cared for free of charge, the father left in a rage.

A few hours later the child returned with a sister. He was crying and exhibited a cut lip and a broken arm. His sister told that he had been beaten for refusing to return and beg for the quarter, and that the first beating had been for swallowing the quarter. The boy was taken into the hospital for treatment of the broken arm. The father appeared later, drunk and abusive, threatening to kill that Doctor Jackson who stole his quarter.

And the doctor will have his personal trials; he is a player in the grand drama. And it may be his patients who supply the humor and equanimity that restore his desponding soul. A Midwestern small-community doctor became disheartened after his fifteen-year-old son crashed a car into a bridge abutment and was killed. The doctor remained at home and answered no calls for two weeks.

Then his patients organized and sent a representative to speak to the doctor. The emissary said, "We share your grief. When we had similar ones you told us we were needed and loved and must continue courageously — and so it is with you. You haven't been in your office for two weeks and things are piling up. We told your nurse to schedule patients for 8 a.m., Monday and we expect you to be there." He was and he didn't miss a day thereafter.

11.

Drugs, Bloodletting and Alcohol

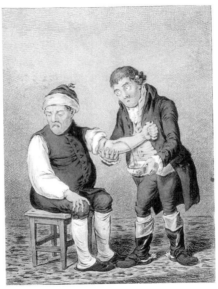

The treatment of afflictions with drugs is a conspicuously droll facet of medicine. In the American Colonies, medicine was folk medicine. The colonists cared for themselves with folk remedies and the colonial governors, clergymen, midwives, apothecaries and self-appointed healers were consulted when home remedies failed to provide relief. Physicians came to the colonies with the first settlers. A surgeon came to Jamestown with Captain John Smith in 1607 and there were four healers aboard the Mayflower when she landed at Plymouth in 1620. But they did not come to practice medicine; they sought to become planters or administrators, and failing this, most of them returned to England.

The colonial governors became medical advisors to their colonies by default. At the Massachusetts Bay Colony, Governor John Winthrop soon was busy advising the sick. He wrote to a doctor in England for a list of currently favored treatments so that he could fulfill the role that was thrust upon him.

But his remedies, even with the benefit of medical advice, rivaled those of a shaman. For smallpox and various obscure fevers, he recommended a drink containing a powder made from pulverized toads. For pain in the breast or in the limbs, he advised wearing a wildcat's skin over the painful part, and for madness, he suggested an herbal tea. The governor's advice was wizardry.

At the Connecticut River Colony, John Winthrop Jr. represented a second generation of healing governors. He was variously an administrator and governor in Connecticut from 1633 to 1676. He did more than simply transmit medical advice, he devised an original panacea. He concocted a drug combination which he called Rubilia. Rubilia was literally a cure for any ailment, and the governor supplied it to ailing colonists for years. Its composition was never revealed. Colonists obtained Rubilia from Winthrop and stored it for future use. When they ran out of it, they wrote for more. It was our first great secret-formula cure-all.

The Connecticut governor also confidently prescribed a drink made by soaking crab eyes in wine, for the relief of bladder stones. And he thought highly of the curative powers of bezoars. Bezoars are concretions — stones — that are formed in the stomachs of various animals. That bezoars can influence the course of disease is a superstition that long antedates the settlement of America. It crossed the ocean in the minds of the colonists and flourished in the New World.

Surely such folly was left behind when the colonies became states and the nation expanded westward. No, it wasn't. Irrational notions have lives of their own. In the 1880s, in our West, boiled toads were highly regarded as a cure for dropsy — heart disease. The skin of a black cat was worn to counter tuberculosis and the entrails of a black cat — killed in the dark of the night — were bound to the heads of persons suffering from epilepsy as a method of treatment. Medical remedies, once they have gained even limited acceptance, endure for incredible periods of time. In 1900 Texans had great confidence in the medical value of bezoars. They put bezoars on snake and mad-dog bites confidently expecting great benefits.

A Texas doctor reported using deer bezoars on ten consecutive cases of mad-dog bites and the bezoars worked in every case.

As the population of the original Colonies increased, clergymen became the communities' healers.

Cotton Mather called the union of theology and healing the Divine Conjunction. It was natural, he said. It was sanctioned by the Almighty. Jesus was a healer — the model.

Mather is our best remembered clergyman-healer. Boston was his domain. He was active there between 1680 and 1726. He was a self-taught healer. Driven by theological impulses, he gathered an immense collection of medical lore through voracious reading.

In the course of his reading, Cotton Mather suffered an experience that medical students have repeated ever since. He developed "fancies that I was myself troubled with almost every Distemper that I read of in my studies; which caused me to use medicines on myself that I might cure my imaginary maladies." Modem medical students commonly develop the symptoms of the diseases they study. It can be a very troubling experience and it may occur several times. One doctor said that in the course of his hospital training he developed the symptoms of almost every disease he studied and that the only place he felt safe was in the obstetrical ward.

Mather wrote a massive medical tome based on his reading. He called it *Angel of Bethesda.*

When he finished it in 1724, he thought that it might well be the most important book ever written. It was to be our first Family Home Medical Encylopedia, but it was never published. We can safely say that nothing was lost.

The clergymen believed that disease was due to sin, and, of course, their prescriptions reflected it. When Mather wrote of consumption (tuberculosis), contrition topped his recommended treatment; "First repent your sins." When he wrote of venereal diseases, the ethereal Divine Conjunction crumbled into ferocious morality. The compassion that healers have been charged to manifest toward the ill since the time of Hippocrates was smothered under revealed righteousness. Of persons afflicted by venereal disease, Mather wrote: "As for any remedies... you are so offensive to me, I'll do nothing for you."

But Puritans were more "earthy" than history has led us to believe. In 1646 there was an outbreak of syphilis in Boston of near epidemic proportions. It was being spread from houses of prostitution.

Among the odd and amusing remedies endorsed by Cotton Mather was one for the treatment of earache. He advised that a roasted turnip — as hot as could be borne — be thrust into the aching ear. One would expect that such a remedy would have a short life, but an analogous remedy, an onion thrust into the ear after boiling, was used for earache on Long Island, New York, in the early 1900s.

There were great expectations that new cures would come from the new plants to be found in the New World and this expectation was shared in Europe. Some fifty plants from the American wilds were touted as valuable new medicinals, among them sassafras, snake root, and peppermint. None ever justified the claims. Teas were made from sassafras blossoms and given for fevers. Wine made from sassafras berries was said to be excellent for colds, and sassafras leaves were applied directly to injuries to stop bleeding.

It is a recurring theme in history that valuable new remedies will be found in new lands — today it is space — or that they will be found in the archives of old lands. We have been examining the ancient remedies of China for the past two hundred years, all without benefit.

In light of this bent of the human psyche, it is not the least surprising that the American colonists looked upon Indian "doctors" favorably and consulted commonly. They were sure that the Indians had secrets.

The popularity of Indian "doctors" has spawned some confusion. The indigenous Indian doctors were herb doctors; their medicinals were made from plants. But very soon some colonists became self-appointed healers and proclaimed that they only used herbs — to set themselves apart from doctors who used medicinals from miscellaneous sources. These colonial healers were also called "Indian doctors." They were widely consulted, but their influence was limited and brief.

On the contrary, the indigenous Indian doctors thrived and have practiced all across the country for two hundred years — they have mystique. The first medical book published in the Midwest was by a clergyman and titled "The Indian Doctor's Depository."

Among other things, the Indians introduced the colonists to tobacco, and in the usual sequence of events, tobacco was endowed with medicinal properties. In the Massachusetts Bay Colony tobacco was taken by mouth for digestive disorders. Inhalation of tobacco smoke was recommended as a remedy for coughing. And tobacco poultices were used to accelerate the healing of wounds.

Cotton Mather wrote that tobacco poured into the ear was good for deafness, and another clergyman-healer advised blowing tobacco smoke into the ear for earache. Mather also lent his authority to the practice of rubbing teeth with the ashes of pipe tobacco to relieve toothache.

One might expect that the Indian enthusiasm for the medicinal value of tobacco would be embraced and then gradually abandoned when it failed — in a rational world perhaps, but not in this one. A hundred years after Mather's time, in 1818, tobacco enemas were touted for the relief of diarrhea. And even after an interval of another hundred years, in 1919, an apparatus for the inflation and fumigation of the colon with tobacco smoke (blown into the intestines by a pump through an enema tube) was popular. It was recommended for constipation or colic. And after an additional half century, accounts of contemporary folk cures in Texas still included blowing tobacco smoke into the ear for earache as well as an inelegant variation that condoned spitting tobacco into the ear for the same affliction.

Clergymen-healers played prominent roles in medical care through the period of the Revolutionary War and the first quarter of the nineteenth century. The Rev. Dr. Joseph Doddridge cared for bodies and souls in western Pennsylvania through the end of this period. His remedies were little changed from those in the colonies two hundred years previously. For erysipelas (a severe facial inflammation) he advised circumscribing the inflamed area with the blood of a black cat. The blood of a black cat was also used in shingles. The blood was obtained by cropping the tail or ears of the cats. As a result there was scarcely a black cat in western Pennsylvania without clipped ears and a shortened tail.

Doddridge advised oil of rattlesnake for rheumatic joints; the flexibility of the snake might be transferable in the oil. It is an ancient Chinese idea still embraced today by those who prefer to believe rather than think.

Healer Doddridge recommended a poultice of roasted turnips for burns and for intestinal purges he gave a drink made by boiling walnut bark in water. The bark was to be peeled downward to effect a diarrheal purge, if vomiting was the desired result, peeling the bark upward could be expected to accomplish this end. Incredible? Of course, but in 1913 — a hundred years later — the residents of eastern North Carolina were peeling elm bark exactly the same way for use in exactly the same manner.

The midwives who delivered our colonial babies did not confine themselves to that practice; they collected folk remedies and applied them for miscellaneous disorders. They treated all the usual children's diseases, and lanced abscessed breasts for nursing mothers. The midwives also made and dispensed pills and salves, and they treated wounds with poultices of corn meal or cow dung.

Cow dung? In Colonial times, folk medicine attributed healing powers to cow dung: it healed boils, it relieved coughing when applied to the chest, and it eased rheumatism if applied to a joint. Sheep dung, chicken and goose dung also had their merits. Surely this practice was so primitive that it could not survive colonial ignorance and superstition.

But it did survive. In 1882 Dr. Francis Long encountered cow dung poultices in Nebraska. Corn huskers used them to "ripen" boils. And in the same period a doctor told of being called to see a girl in Vermont who had suffered extensive burns. He found her covered with a one-half inch layer of hen manure, and relatives declined to remove it when he protested.

Were these eccentric, last-gasp examples — the type that can always be found if one is determined to make a lurid case? Not quite. In 1900, George King found that "cow flop" poultices were in common use on Long Island, New York. And in 1910 Dr. Joseph Jerger, who practiced in Waterloo, Iowa, was called to a rural home to see a boy suffering with measles and pneumonia. He found the child covered with steaming fresh cow manure, and the manure was covered with a tarpaulin to contain the heat.

Colonial midwives — and doubtless other contemporary practitioners — also credited a human excretory product with medicinal value: urine. Human urine was taken by mouth mixed with a sweetener, honey, for instance. It was recommended for sore throats, rheumatism, consumption, and as a mouth wash to preserve teeth and prevent mouth odor.

Urine therapy has an ultra-ancient history. There are records of the ingestion of urine for disease in Chinese annals of the third century B.C. Do ancient Chinese remedies have an element of immortality or are they reinvented? In California in the 1850s, fresh urine poured into the ear was a widely known remedy for earache and in the Ozarks in the 1930s it was given to children, mixed with a sweetener, for digestive ailments. American medical folklore also asserts that washing one's face with the wet diaper of a newborn prevents and removes freckles. For an update, in 1970 when researchers reported that urine contains an enzyme that might be useful in the treatment of phlebitis, people wrote in to thank them for proving that it was beneficial to consume urine.

The clergymen, midwives and miscellaneous healers of the pre-Revolutionary War period also prescribed remedies made from chimney soot, sow bugs (wood lice) and bedbugs. Bear grease, since it was from an agile animal, was used as a remedy for rheumatism.

With such remedies in general use, there would seem to be no room for quack doctors. But designing minds are endlessly inventive and quackery got off to an early start in the Colonies. In 1737 a letter in a Boston newspaper told of "Shoemakers, Weavers, and Almanac makers... who have laid aside the proper business of their lives to turn Quacks." And in 1757 a history of New York related that quacks "abound like locusts in Egypt." Grocers, tailors, postmasters and booksellers all sold medical remedies.

"Bitters" were the favorite remedies offered by the quacks. Bitters were simply bitter liquids. The more bitter they were, the better they were thought to be.

Quacks vied with one another to devise drinks of unequaled bitterness. They were said to be good for everything, but especially for fevers. Bitters were analogous to quinine which was discovered in Peru about 1630 and brought to Europe about 1633. Quinine was very good for malarial fever and it was very bitter.

Bitters were made from sarsaparilla, snake root, squaw mint and dogwood, usually extracts, in alcohol. In our western mountain states in the 1800s, bitters were represented by a drink made of one-quarter pint of buffalo gall (the secretion of the gall bladder of a buffalo) mixed with a pint of water. Gall is exceedingly bitter. These preparations were swallowed in punishing amounts when fever struck.

The idea that bitter medicine is the best medicine has a large following and a venerable tradition.

Oliver Wendell Holmes wrote: "The popular belief is all but universal that sick people should feed on noxious substances."

By 1776 there were some four hundred doctors in the Colonies with degrees from foreign medical schools. It was the beginning of medical progress in the Colonies, but it was only a beginning. Alexander Hamilton, a Scot, graduated from medical school in Edinburgh and arrived in America in 1739. He described the doctors of Albany, New York. They were all self-taught; they absorbed folklore and superstition; they studied herbs and kept shops in which they sold drugs. Hamilton thought that medicine in Albany was "a mean thing and unworthy of the application of a gentleman."

He described how the healing trade gained a new member. A very good shoemaker was somehow thought to have cured a woman of "a pestilent mortal disease," and as a result was applied to by ill persons from all quarters. "Finding the practice of physic a more profitable business than cobbling soles, he fell to cobbling human bodies."

The new healers, the European-trained doctors, had primitive concepts of the nature of disease.

They thought that disease was caused by imbalances of the body's natural equilibrium — excesses or depletions of vague body "humours" — and that it was to be combated vigorously by purges, pukes, sweats, clysters (enemas), blistering, and bleeding — interventions that would restore the equilibrium of the humours.

Everyone who was ill was to be purged. Calomel was the favorite purgative. It was a violent drug, so violent that patients who had been subjected to it feared repeating the experience. They wrote verses about the doctors' unbridled use of it. This one appeared in a Richmond, Virginia, paper:

Howe'er their patients do complain
Of head or heart or nerve or vein
Of fevers thirsts or temper fell
The medicine still is Calomel.
And they prayed to be spared, as in this verse:
And when I must resign my breath
Pray let me die a natural death
And bid you all a long farewell
Without one dose of Calomel.

The subject lent itself to black humor. A story circulated about a doctor who had given a large dose of calomel to a patient who was mortally ill. The next morning he inquired if the purgative had worked. "Yes indeed," he was told. "Ten times before he died and nine times afterward."

A few doctors soon became skeptical of the value of calomel and a few saw the public's apprehension as an opportunity.

About 1820 a practitioner opening an office in Indiana put up a sign "Joseph S. Burr, root doctor, no calomel." And in Michigan a doctor advertised that he could "cure any curable disease more successfully without calomel than any doctor can with it."

Bloodletting was another treatment that early doctors applied in almost every significant illness.

It was common to lance an arm vein and encourage the blood to flow until the patient was about to faint.

The usual amount of blood taken was twelve ounces. But Dr. Samuel Gross, professor of surgery at the Cincinnati Medical College, knew well the bent of the public mind. In

1840 he wrote that he usually took sixteen to twenty-four ounces of blood because his patients did not seem to think they were getting their money's worth if he took less.

And the public was so generally persuaded to the value of bloodletting that it was common practice for people to visit their doctor in the spring and again in the fall for a routine bloodletting. It "cleansed the blood" and thereby perpetuated good health and protected one from disease. Bloodletting was practiced throughout the eighteenth century in America and though it began to decline after 1825, it was not uncommon as late as 1875.

Leeches were sold by apothecaries for do-it-yourself bloodletting and if need be one could employ a "leech man," who was said to able to get a leech to bite when others could not. One leech can draw about an ounce of blood in an hour. The leeches were collected from rivers and even imported from Europe.

Vomiting, usually induced by ipecac, was another standard measure used by doctors to fight disease by balancing the humours.

When they recorded the administration of ipecac, doctors wrote, "I puked her," or "I gave her a puke." Ipecac has a penetrating scent. It shrouded the doctor in an identifying mantle that Oliver Wendell Holmes said was commonly so strong that just having the doctor pass through a sick chamber released a sufficient dose of the drug.. Elsewhere people recognized a doctor by this peculiar fragrance.

The apothecary shops stocked countless odd remedies — all of them useless. Daniel Drake described a typical shop in the 1870s as stocked with numerous paper bundles of herbs, bottles partly stopped with eroded corks and open jars of ointments releasing a multitude of fragrances and possessing a potential effectiveness "not a whit behind those of the apothecary in the time of Solomon." Ginseng and garlic would have been prominent, and they have survived.

But even in Colonial times, astute observers — even

some who were not doctors — knew that most of this medical practice was delusional. Benjamin Franklin wrote, "He's the best physician who knows the worthlessness of most medicines."

In 1860 Dr. Holmes thought that mankind would be better off if all of the drugs then available were sunk to the bottom of the sea — but he feared that the fishes would suffer. And later he remarked that no families take so little medicine as those of doctors, except those of apothecaries.

As the twentieth century dawned, nothing had changed. Dr. Osier at Johns Hopkins, the greatest physician-teacher of his day, often quoted Holmes on drugs. And Osier wrote that the desire to take medicine was the most distinguishing difference between men and animals. He asserted that one of the prime duties of a physician is to educate his patients not to take medicine. Osier well knew the power of suggestion and the ease with which men delude themselves. Tongue in cheek, he advised doctors that when a new drug came out they should treat all of their patients with it immediately — before it lost its effectiveness.

The tale is told of the doctor who mixed up the prescriptions of an elderly patient and his wife. Each of them was delighted with the new medicine and both of them were cured.

When doctors finally dosed less, the public increased its purchases of patent medicines and dosed itself more. Patent medicines were imported from England early in the eighteenth century and were very popular after 1750. A ship arriving at Philadelphia in 1759 carried Anderson's Pills, Squire's Elixir, Bostock's Elixir, Lokyer's Pills, British Oil and Stoughton's Bitters. All were advertised for immediate sale.

American originals appeared very shortly and got a great boost when the Revolutionary War cut off the British supply. Swain's Panacea was a popular one. Swain was a bookbinder turned medical entrepreneur. His panacea was advertised to cure tuberculosis, sore throats, rheumatism, bone disease, syphilis and bad livers. There was also Shinn's Panacea and a Porter's Vegetable Catholicum, which were said to cure a similar group of afflictions. Many of these nostrums were 15-30 percent alcohol, which greatly enhanced their appeal. Newspapers and almanacs carried an increasing volume of advertising for such products through the first half of the nineteenth century.

After the Civil War, patent medicine quackery entered its Golden Age. Many doctors abetted the fraud. They prescribed the products and countenanced the advertising even in medical journals. Peruna was the best known of the deceptive patent medicines and it became the most recognized trade name in the nation.

It was created by Dr. Samuel Hartman, who graduated from the Jefferson Medical College in 1857. It was good for everything. Hartman said that all diseases were caused by catarrh, and that Peruna cured catarrh. Fifty members of Congress endorsed it. A 30 percent alcohol content assured its popularity. The same feature caused the government to ban its sale on Indian reservations and the IRS was moved to put a liquor sales tax on it.

Dr. Ezra Michener told how at the beginning of the nineteenth century at the age of six, "I became a would-be drunkard." He suffered frequently from stomach colic, so his mother dosed him with various patent medicines until "such was the appetite I acquired for alcohol in almost any form that more then four score years of abstinence have hardly abated its intensity."

And a dean of Duke University's School of Medicine recalled how as a boy in 1906 he explored his grandfather's attic and found it filled with empty patent medicine bottles, including Lydia Pinkham's Vegetable Compound — a notably alcoholic nostrum. His grandfather was a strict prohibitionist. Did he know what he was consuming? Probably not, but it was clear from the number of bottles that he consumed it with great relish. Others did know and bought it for precisely that reason.

At the turn of the century, *Collier's Magazine* and *The Ladies Home Journal* exposed the patent medicine fraud. Samuel Hopkins Adams wrote that, "It would take nearly nine bottles of beer to put as much alcohol into a thirsty man's system as a temperance advocate can get by drinking one bottle of Hostetter's Stomach Bitters."

After two hundred years of enthusiasm for drugs in America, there were fewer than six that could be regarded as having any demonstrable value. In 1938, sulfanilamide was discovered and the modern era of scientific study and application of drugs was born. Maturation was slow and irregular. There was a romance with vitamin C to be endured, as well as bizarre cures for cancer — Laetrile, of course, and shark cartilage in 1996. No doubt such things will continue, but science is in the saddle.

Alcohol has the distinction of having provided more pleasure and more pain than any other substance consumed by mankind. In the American Colonies alcohol was ubiquitous. Men downed a bracing dram of rum, whisky, or brandy on awakening in the morning; an abstemious man might limit himself to a mug of cider. Beer and cider or spirits mixed with water were part of every meal. Water was regarded suspiciously (with some justification because water sources were often contaminated). Fermented or distilled preparations were thought to be better for one's health.

The first distillery in Boston was opened in 1700. At the turn of the eighteenth century Americans consumed more alcohol than any other people on earth. Farmers took a jug with them into the fields and paused for mid-morning and mid-afternoon refreshment. Bottles passed freely at social gatherings where imbibing from them was referred to as "kissing Black Betty." Clergymen imbibed without prejudice — unless they fumbled the Sunday sermon as a result. Midwives dispensed alcohol freely to alleviate the pains of childbirth. And doctors expected to "have a drop" at each house they visited — before seeing the patient.

Doctors who drank recklessly were widely regarded as the best doctors, providing their services were engaged early in the day when moderate stimulation supposedly enabled them to prescribe with extraordinary insight. Physicians' indulgence raised criticism only if it was extreme. A physician who came to Maryland in 1638 was shortly thereafter charged with flagrant intemperance, but a witness on his behalf testified that he was not so drunk that he couldn't get out of a cart's way — apparently an exonerating defense.

Whisky was referred to as "conversation fluid." If a doctor took on just what was called a "talking load," patients might react quite favorably. Oliver Wendell Holmes recorded the attitude of an Irish laborer when he asked the Irishman about his doctor, who was well known to be overly fond of spirits: "I like him best when he's a little that way," the Irishman replied. "Then I can spake to him."

In Illinois, Dr. Charles Johnson told of a colleague who was "utterly besotted with long drinking." The confidence of his patients was so great that they did not wait for him to sober up. If he was needed when he was dead drunk, he was located, put in a wagon and hauled "like a dead hog" to the home of the patient, where time would be given him to sober up. Then he would be taken to the patient, his diagnosis received with great confidence and his recommended treatment carried out with absolute faithfulness.

Occasionally a temperate community insisted on a temperate doctor. In 1796 the people of Troy, New Hampshire, bargained with a doctor who moved there. He was known for alcoholism. The community bought a horse and medicines for him in return for a pledge that he would abstain for a year. He left at the end of the year.

If an inebriated doctor attended an intemperate patient and tragedy was avoided, comedy was certain to ensue. An old tale of uncertain locale tells of a doctor summoned to a lady's bedside when his thought processes were much blunted by spirits. He began his examination by counting her pulse, and when he lost track of the count he tried again. He lost track of the count again and on a third effort he fared no better. "Drunk, by God," he said, and terminated the visit with a quick exit.

The next morning the doctor considered the ways to repair the damage: How to explain his behavior? The woman involved was a respected person and a valued patient. As he was mulling the matter, a note was delivered to his desk. The woman was as worried as he was. She wrote to apologize for bothering him and entreated him to keep her indisposition a secret.

For a time alcohol was considered to have medicinal value. It was erroneously regarded as a stimulant and in some areas it was the most widely prescribed medicine. And it was often prescribed heroically.

In 1807 during an epidemic of meningitis in Connecticut one physician prescribed two quarts of brandy and one quart of wine to be taken in the course of twenty-four hours. A gallon of whisky might be given in twenty-four hours. Whisky was thought to be good for dyspepsia in some quarters, and three pints of rye whisky "purified the blood." The records do not inform us about the results.

Some habitues claimed other merits for alcohol. A man who fell off his front porch and broke his arm told his doctor: "Damn it, I was sober as a judge when I fell. If I'd been drunk it never would have happened."

As the toxic effects of alcohol became evident, physicians came to advise against its use and to some degree follow their own advice. They also devised maxims to be followed when a patient's consumption of alcohol was being appraised: "A man's claim regarding the use of alcohol should be doubled, a woman's tripled or quadrupled, and a teetotaler's entirely discounted." A Scotch doctor defined four stages of drunkenness: Jocose, Bellicose, Lacrimose and Comatose. These correspond roughly to another description, said to be an oriental proverb, that "One glass of wine makes a man into a lion, two, into a rabbit, three into a monkey and four into a swine."

To their patients, doctors repeated aphorisms such as "Drunkenness is voluntary insanity," and "Alcohol is the devil in solution." Tipplers countered with a few aphorisms of their own, such as: "The brewery is the best drugstore," and "There are more old drunkards than old doctors." And wags had fun with the issue;

> *Pure water is the best of gifts*
> *That gods to man can bring*
> *But who am I that I should have*
> *The best of anything?*
> *Let monarchs gather round the pump*
> *And pass the dipper free;*
> *But whisky, rum, or even wine*
> *Is good enough for me.*

When hospitals came into being, particularly the charity hospitals, alcoholism and its multitude of complications was the most common affliction they were called upon to treat. Many patients were deathly ill; many were simply drunk, but they were helpless and without support or assistance. The hospitals took them in.

Resident doctors reacted to the tide of alcoholics entering their hospitals, particularly alcoholics who came in repeatedly and used the hospital as a sanctuary for recovery. The alcoholics took up an inordinate amount of the doctors' time and they took up beds that were in demand for other patients.

In the 1940s and 1950s, the Boston City Hospital, which served and employed the Irish of Boston, was a Mecca for alcoholics. Whole wards if not the whole hospital had an "ambiance of muscatel." An overworked resident protested. These were not afflictions of nature, this was self-indulgence, in the same category as mugging, larceny, and murder. And another distraught resident proclaimed loudly that alcoholism

was an "ethnic disease belonging to the Irish." Unfortunately
he proclaimed it in the dining room of the hospital. A month
passed before any waitress would serve him again.

The care and treatment of alcoholics is probably the
ultimate test of a doctor's sense of humor. Prevarication and
duplicity complicate the task to a degree that would be intolerable if the ingenuity demonstrated simultaneously was
not so impressive. To cache alcohol in a hospital requires
inventiveness of top quality. One innovative convalescent
tippler hid his secret bottle in the reservoir of his toilet. This
worked for a while, but the bottle ultimately moved to block
the cut-off mechanism in the water reservoir and the overflow
flooded the room, the corridors and the room below. It was
a disaster, but for the doctor it was just another droll facet
of alcoholism.

And despite the view of some that alcoholics are born
unhappy, they contribute a great deal of saving humor to the
medical scene. One sick man in an alcoholic delirium pulled
an intravenous feeding needle out of the vein in his arm. As a
result blood flowed out freely and soaked the sheets. The poor
fellow had enough presence of mind to clasp the arm firmly
with his opposite hand to stanch the flow of blood.

When a resident doctor arrived to rescue the situation
the patient said, "Gee, I'm glad to see you. I'm giving this
fellow first aid."

12.

Surgeons

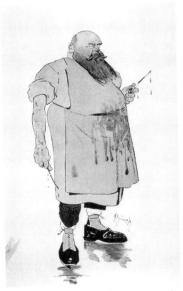

Surgeons are self-confident, dexterous, decisive and diligent. The challenge of the endeavor soon eliminates those
who are not. Their self-esteem inflates easily to hubris. Most
surgeons come to believe that, in their niche, they are the best.
It is said to be every surgeon's tragedy that when he requires
surgery the man with the greatest skill will not be available.

And there are tales to justify such hubris. In 1911 Dr.
Charles Mayo, the younger of the famous brothers, was suddenly taken ill while in New York. He diagnosed his affliction
as an inflamed gall bladder, but the surgeons who were called
to attend him thought that it was appendicitis. Surgery was

undertaken and Dr. Mayo's appendix was removed. Within a few days his condition deteriorated to a degree that raised fears for his life. New York newspapers reported that he was dying. On re-evaluation, the attending surgeons concluded that Dr. Mayo did indeed need gall bladder surgery; a prompt second operation to remove his gall bladder restored his health.

Dr. Mayo's diagnostic skill was superb, but surgery teaches humility to the best of surgeons — and surgeons know it. They come to treasure tales of inglorious encounters because it is the challenge and attraction of surgery that frustration comes repeatedly from the most unexpected quarters and that mastery is always just beyond one's grasp. A surgeon's tale of how he was humbled is much more interesting to his fellows than any account of his success.

A Philadelphia surgeon of the 1920s told how exaltation can be followed by dejection and dismay in the course of a few minutes. On his morning hospital round an elderly woman whom he treated successfully grasped his hand, kissed it and murmured in reverent tones, "Second only to God." The surgeon wrote: "This seemed to be a somewhat generous, but satisfactory appraisal and I proceeded to the out-patient department on light wings."

In the out-patient department he was appointed to see a man he had operated upon a few weeks previously. This patient was an emaciated, dour looking fellow. And when the surgeon inquired, "How are you?" the man responded bitterly. "You ruined me!" he said.

Abashedness, when it comes, may be self-induced. Dr. William Halstead, a contemporary of the Mayo brothers, was surgeon-in-chief at the prestigious Johns Hopkins Hospital. Dr. Halstead developed intermittent, severe chest pain and diagnosed his affliction as heart disease. At times the pain forced him to leave the operating room and turn his surgery over to an assistant. Halstead did not consult his medical colleagues; what could they tell him that he didn't already know? He suffered on until he finally developed jaundice which made it obvious that his pain was coming from his gall bladder instead of his heart, and that he needed surgery.

A few surgeons evaded submission when they required surgery. Dr. Evan Kane of Pennsylvania, took out his own appendix when he was sixty years old — the first surgeon ever to do so. And when he was seventy he operated on himself successfully for a hernia.

In colonial America surgery was limited to external procedures such as amputation of a limb or a breast, removal of surface growths, opening of abscesses, and to a few shallow invasive procedures such as removal of stones from the urinary bladder or freeing a strangulated hernia. Speed was essential inasmuch as anesthesia, blood transfusions and other supportive measures were unknown and patients almost always died if an operation was not concluded quickly. Successful surgeons were noted for their swiftness and many anecdotes were related to recall a given surgeon's celerity.

Surgery was performed in homes. There was only one public general hospital in America before the Revolutionary War and fewer than one hundred at the time of the Civil War. Spectators gathered in the houses to watch the operations and one account describes how they "filled the open doors and windows."

Another account tells of spectators watching through the windows of a street-level room. In this instance the surgeon invited two of them in, one to assist him and other to hold a lamp. The assistant soon became giddy and had to leave. The spectators timed the operations and compared one surgeon's performance time with another's.

When the first limb amputation was performed in Philadelphia, in 1699, speed played a vital role in its success: "As the arm was cut off, some spirits in a basin happened to take fire, and being spilt on the surgeon's apron, set his clothes on fire — but running into the street, the fire was quenched; and so quick was the surgeon's return that the patient had not lost very much blood, though left in that open bleeding condition." This surgeon was fast with his feet as well as his hands — and spectators had partially obstructed his flight.

An early account of a leg amputation related that the leg was "on the floor" in one minute and forty seconds, and the bleeding vessels were tied and the wound dressed inside of three minutes.

Of another surgeon it was said that he was so swift that on one occasion, with one sweep of his knife, he had cut off the limb of his patient, three fingers of his assistant, and the coat-tails of a spectator.

Experienced observers were said to advise newcomers at some operations not to blink — they might miss the operation. And a Texas surgeon of the 1850s was described as so swift and dexterous that "he could shave a running jackrabbit."

These feats were performed in home kitchens into the twentieth century. Kitchens were selected because they were usually the largest room in a house and had the sturdiest tables. The walls and floor were scrubbed before the operation and a wet sheet might be tacked to the ceiling over the table to keep off any dust. A kerosene lamp or candles provided the light, and family members moved them about when light at special angle was required.

Kitchen surgery had some unique problems and complications. A Midwestern surgeon told of being in the middle of an operation on a woman weighing three hundred pounds when the kitchen table began to sag and threatened to collapse. The surgeon directed a male member of the family to get under the table on his hands and knees and to hold the table up with his back. The operation was completed with the man under the table protesting loudly that he could not continue much longer.

Late in the nineteenth century a Baltimore surgeon was called to a small town to perform an emergency abdominal operation. He selected and positioned a table for surgery leaving just enough room for himself on one side and for the local doctor, acting as his assistant, on the other side. Just as the doctors were ready to begin, a stout woman, a friend of the patient, appeared and said that she had promised to be at the patient's side and she intended to keep her promise. She was adamant, so she was allowed to pass to the head of the table where she could see everything and the doctors began the operation.

The insistent friend soon felt ill and decided that she must step out. But there was no passage on either side of the table.

The surgeon suggested that she crawl under the table — but she must not on her life jar the table.

She tried. Her shoulders passed between the legs of the table, but her hips would not go, and she was stuck!

The surgeon admonished her — she must not jar the table — and kept her there for a quarter of an hour, until it was safe to pause a moment and step aside while the unfortunate woman worked herself backward and then rushed from the room. In rural areas some surgeons preferred to operate outside of the house — in the yard. The light was better, there was plenty of room for those who came to watch, and they could be made to stand back more easily. Dr. Herff, practicing in western Texas in the 1840s, told how he waited for a day that was cloud free and dustless, and how he stationed a dozen persons around the operating table with palm fans to keep the flies away.

Most surgeons picked a site under a large tree for their outdoor surgery. One expressed a decided preference for an apple tree. He said that he had never had an infection in an operation performed under an apple tree. In the South, outdoor operations were still common in the early 1900s.

The scope of surgery expanded rapidly after Dr. Crawford W. Long, a Georgian, discovered that ether induced a state of senselessness that permitted surgery without pain. The first public demonstration of the effectiveness of ether took place at the Massachusetts General Hospital in Boston in

October 1846.

A photographer was brought in to record the great occasion, but he was so unnerved by the blood that flowed that he had to leave before he got a picture.

Ether anesthesia generated some marvelous surgical comedies. Dr. John C. Warren, the surgeon who performed the first operation under ether, participated in a hilarious ether imbroglio. Dr. Warren planned to operate on an athletic young man who became very excited as he was being put to sleep. Ether induces a sense of elation, and it is common for this to rise to a wild excitement before unconsciousness occurs. The young man struggled to rise up as he was being put to sleep and, though several resident doctors hastened to restrain him, he rolled off the operating table knocking over the candle stands that were the source of illumination. The doctors grappled with the patient in the darkness under the table where he seemed to double his resistance. But he was finally subdued and held spread-eagle while the anesthetist clamped the ether mask to his face again and poured ether generously until heavy breathing indicated that the patient was finally asleep. When the lamps were lit, the patient was seen cowering in a corner and one of the residents was on the floor sleeping soundly under the ether mask.

The excitement induced by ether was such that four or five persons might be required to restrain a muscular patient and sometimes four or five persons were not immediately available. In San Antonio, before there was a hospital, Dr. Ferdinand Herff sometimes operated in a hotel room on patients who came in from outlying areas. He once used ether in a case of a herculean man who had a massive growth on his back between his shoulder blades. Dr. Herff had two stalwart porters on hand to hold the patient down if he became excited. But the precaution was inadequate. As the incision was made the patient leaped off the table, ran down a stairway, dashed across the hotel lobby into an outdoor plaza trailing blood from a partially removed tumor flapping on his back; and with two doctors and the sturdy porters running after him. The patient fell in the plaza where he was pinned down while Dr. Herff completed the operation with two swift strokes and then threw a towel over the wound. They carried the patient back into the hotel and Dr. Herff put in some closing stitches. The result was perfect.

If a patient submitted to ether quietly, there might be some comical vocalizing before sleep ensued. At Johns Hopkins, Dr. Hugh Young, subsequently a world famous urologist, often served as an anesthetist when he was a resident. On one occasion he gave ether to a young lady who was to have an operation in a large amphitheater before a group of doctors gathered for a surgical seminar. Just as his patient went to sleep, she rolled her eyes at him and murmured, "Kiss me again, Dr. Young." Her appeal was loud enough to be easily heard by the spectators and Dr. Young was embarrassed. "If she just hadn't said *again,*" he complained.

In rural settings, whoever was available might be pressed into service as the anesthetist — under the surgeon's direction of course. A surgeon told how in one instance he had a mother give ether as he did an appendectomy on her son and on another occasion he amputated a man's leg while the patient's wife administered the anesthetic. In isolated locations emergencies called for heroic actions. Another surgeon told of operating on a pool table in a poolroom-barbershop with the barber giving the anesthetic and on another occasion operating in a market with his patient on a butcher block and the butcher giving the anesthetic.

The effect of ether wears off quickly. Patients might rouse up in the course of an operation, and if not given more ether promptly, they might disrupt the procedure in various ways. In the 1800s, most houses had wood shingle roofs. Fires were much feared. A cry of "Fire!" caused great alarm and set off all kinds of emergency responses. In this era a Baltimore surgeon was required to operate in an outlying village, at a home, in a room on the second floor. It was a warm summer day and all of the windows were open. The patient, who had an abscess on his posterior, was only lightly anesthetized for safety, He was drowsy, but not deeply asleep.

The surgeon had need to cauterize a bit of tissue (touch it lightly with a hot iron to stop bleeding) and when he did, the patient felt a sting and an odor of burnt flesh tainted the air. The patient aroused immediately and shouted "Fire" with an intensity that seemed likely to carry for several blocks and galvanize all of the town's volunteer firefighters. The doctors tried to stuff a towel in the patient's mouth, but that made him double his efforts to call out. Then they closed the windows.

Infection was the first barrier to expanding the use of surgery. The first innovation to prevent infection came in 1865. It involved spraying operating room, the patient, and the surgeon with carbolic acid. Carbolic acid killed bacteria and surgical infections were dramatically reduced. Puckish surgeons of that period began their operations with an order mimicking an invocation: "Let us spray," they said.

The Johns Hopkins Hospital was the first to garb its surgeons in white cotton shirts and trousers — to be worn under their operating gowns — and it also supplied them with white caps. It was a measure to reduce the chances that bacteria might enter the operating room on clothing or hair.

Shortly after this practice began, Dr. Howard Kelly was in surgery when he was informed that a woman scheduled for surgery on the following day had been admitted to the hospital. At the conclusion of his operation, Dr. Kelly walked to her room and chatted with her briefly to refresh his memory of her problem, then he returned to his operating room. The woman summoned a nurse immediately — she was indignant, "A fine sort of institution," she protested. "The cook has just been in and asked me some very impertinent questions!"

In 1886 Dr. Reginald Fitz in Boston recognized and described how appendicitis took lives and how this toll could be eliminated by surgery. With anesthesia and a means to combat infection available, the great age of surgery began — the growth of hospitals and the era of great surgeons, Dr. Halstead in Baltimore, the Mayo brothers in Minnesota, Dr. Charles Frazier of Philadelphia, Drs. J.P. Murphy and Christian Fenger in Chicago, and Dr. Crile in Cleveland, to mention a few. These surgeons led demanding lives because it was their credo that the patient's welfare was paramount and that no demand that contributed to that end was too great to be met. A surgeon came by definition to be one who is "worried about the past, anxious about the future and up to his neck in present troubles."

Dr. Arthur Allen, a principal surgeon at the Massachusetts General Hospital in the 1930s and '40s personified the dedicated surgeon and he accepted the continuous perturbation that is part of a surgeon's life. He said that the surgeon who didn't awaken at 2 a.m. and worry for an hour did not deserve to be a surgeon. When Dr. Allen arrived at the hospital in the morning, his first question to his resident was always, "What's the bad news?"

Four or more persons standing toe to toe around an operating table is a situation with potential for comedy, especially when there is a hierarchical portioning of the available space. At Johns Hopkins, Dr. Halstead was a remote, austere man with infinite patience. His patience was exemplified on one occasion when near the end of a long operation, he said to an assistant: "Would you mind moving a little? You've been standing on my foot for the last half hour."

Patience governed Halstead's great contribution to surgery. He insisted on delicate and meticulous handling of the tissues. With anesthesia, speed was no longer primary. This prolonged his operating time and some of his fellow surgeons thought that his delicacy was overdone. A "Halstead" became a synonym for an interminable operation. Dr. William Mayo joked that by the time Dr. Halstead put in the last stitch, the incision was healed. But Halstead had made a very important point and it changed surgery.

Other surgeons were less patient than Dr. Halstead when there was competition for floor space. In Philadelphia of the 1930s, neurosurgeon Charles Frazier used thick pads of gauze about the size of washcloths in his operations. An assistant told how one of the pads once slipped to the floor. He watched it go and then he stepped on it. Neurosurgical operations are often very long and there are periods when an assistant has nothing to do. In such moments this assistant sought out the pad on the floor with his foot and "amused myself by rocking on it and pressing the fluid out of it."

As the operation progressed, "the Old Man got more and more restless and his elbows began to jerk." The assistant moved away a bit because Dr. Frazier was known to give assistants some very hard blows to the ribs when his elbows began to jerk. It was a sign that he was becoming irritated. "But I kept my foot on the sponge," the assistant said. And he continued:" Suddenly Pop threw down his instruments and said, 'My God! Who's stamping on my foot?'" The assistant wrote, "It was the best moment of my week."

He was pleased because surgeons commonly harass and abuse their assistants. Some do it to relieve their tensions, some think it is the way to teach, and a few are just plain nasty. Residents come to savor a little retribution no matter what its source or form.

One exhausted and angry resident, at the end of a trying day in the operating room, penned the common situation in a verse titled "The Swearing Surgeon." In part it reads:

I try his every whim to satisfy
But, so it seems, the more I do
The more he growls — and curses, too
At everyone he's bound to swear
That lap sheet isn't folded right
This scalpel's dull!
Those ties won't hold
For Christ's sake weren't you nurses told

How many Mayo clamps I need,
When something major starts to bleed?
For God's sake, Doctor, cut that tie!
Don't stand there gazing at the sky!

Surgeons were sometimes abashed by their own behavior and the tensions it left behind. Boston surgeon Maurice Richardson expressed it when John Homans was his assistant: "What I like about you John is that after a difficult operation you always speak to me the next day. Some of my assistants haven't been willing to speak to me for several days."

Dr. Ernest Sachs, the first professor of neurosurgery at Washington University in St. Louis, chattered during his operations. He harassed his assistants continuously with denigrating pleas implying that they were both obtuse and inept. His common line during an operation was, "Help me, help me, will someone please help me?"

On one celebrated occasion he was operating with only local anesthesia — skin anesthesia at the operative site, but the patient is awake — contrary to his usual practice. It was a late night emergency and the circumstances made him more irascible than usual. Very shortly he forgot the nature of the anesthesia and launched into his usual chatter, "Help me, help me," and the frequency and bite of his taunts increased as the operation progressed. As the surgeons petulance reached a peak, "Help me, help me please," a weak voice issued from beneath the surgical drapes — it was the patient: "Won't somebody please help Dr. Sachs? Don't let me die."

Dr. John Homans was also a voluble surgeon. At least one patient had doubts that he could talk continuously and operate well at the same time. On that occasion Homans was garrulous while doing a hemorrhoidectomy under local anesthesia and his patient spoke up. "Doctor Homans," he said. "More work and less talk, please."

But a surgeon of grave deportment might also generate comedy in the operating room. Dr. Howard Kelly at the Johns

Hopkins Hospital was a profoundly religious man who prayed with some of his patients both before and after surgery. He sometimes thought it appropriate to kneel beside the operating table and pray as the anesthetic was about to be given to his patient. This was comforting to some patients, but it terrified others. The anesthetists sometimes begged that prayers be postponed until after surgery. A patient agitated by fear of surgery might be pushed to such a state of terror by prayer that it was virtually impossible to put him to sleep.

In Detroit Dr. Frederick Schreiber told of a surgeon who prayed with a patient in his room and asked God's help in the next morning's operation. The patient promptly cancelled the surgery. He said: "If you need that much help, I need another surgeon."

Identification of patients in an operating room is a very serious matter. Misidentification has led to some great tragedies. But, of course, the subject has a humorous side. At the University of Michigan a woman who required rectal surgery asked that it be done by Dr. Frederick Coller, who was the professor of surgery for a quarter of a century beginning in 1930. She said that he had operated on her before. The surgical resident informed Dr. Coller, who said he did not remember the woman and doubted that he had seen her before, but gave the resident permission to add the case to the next morning's busy schedule. When he entered the operating room the next morning the woman was already asleep and draped for surgery with only her buttocks exposed to view. Dr. Coller glanced at the exposed posterior as he donned his gloves and said, "Nope, never saw her before in my life."

Dedicated, driving surgeons find it hard to tolerate reticence in others who care for the sick. The story is told of an ardent neurosurgeon who visited a hospital patient and found him on a bedpan. The surgeon removed the bedpan and offered it to an orderly who was in the room emptying a wastebasket. The orderly declined to accept it and said it wasn't his job to empty bedpans. Asked what his job was, he said he cleaned floors. The surgeon turned the bedpan upside down, emptied the contents on the floor, dropped the bedpan in the middle of the puddle and told the orderly to get a mop and clean the floor.

When patients declined to accept their advice, surgeons of yesteryear sometimes sought ways to compel compliance. They would find a way to make a patient do what was good for him. The integrity of doctors was such that family, friends, and even the clergy might connive with a surgeon to accomplish what was thought necessary.

Dr. Farrar Cobb opened a surgical practice in Boston in 1890. He was called to see a woman hospitalized for abdominal distress, and he found that she had an intestinal obstruction. Dr. Cobb advised surgery, but the lady refused. He told her that she would surely die, but still she refused.

Dr. Cobb sought help from the clergy, but his patient was unmoved by a visit of a priest. The earnest priest took a chained cross from his neck, held it over her and said, "I command you in the name of God and the holy pope of Rome to submit to the operation." Her response was to strike the cross from his hand and rage, "To hell with you and the pope."

The priest asked Dr. Cobb if he was sure the lady would die. Dr. Cobb said it was a certainty. "Very well," said the priest, and while an attendant held the patient, the priest held an ether mask to her face until she was anesthetized. Then the priest fainted away.

Today's surgeons rely on persuasion. Some are very adept at it. At the University of Michigan, Dr. Coller did many operations for cancer of the intestinal tract which required the creation of a colostomy. A colostomy is an opening through the skin on the lower abdomen which serves as a permanent rectum after the surgery. Patients who were depressed when they learned they had cancer sometimes lost heart completely when they contemplated life with a colostomy. Dr. Coller could erase depression and restore hope. He said: "Now if the good Lord had originally placed your rectum upon your abdomen, and I came along and said, 'My man, you have a problem that I can only correct by putting your rectum down between your legs,' you would say to me, 'Hell, that's an awful place to put my rectum — between my legs.' Now, my man, I'm going to put your rectum in a convenient place on your abdomen where you can see it easily without having to get a mirror, where you can keep it clean and watch it function every day."

His residents said that Dr. Coller was so persuasive that they sometimes wondered if they shouldn't have their rectums changed.

Sometimes a harmless ruse will induce prompt patient compliance with a doctor's directions. Dr. Eustace Sloop practiced in rural North Carolina where he made calls to scattered farmhouses and sometimes encountered situations that he was not well-equipped to handle. On one rural call in the early 1900s he found a boy with a gaping facial laceration that extended across his forehead and into his scalp. Dr. Sloop had only ordinary suture material in his bag. The stitches required would leave a permanent disfiguring scar if he used it, but if very fine sutures were used the scar could be much reduced.

Dr. Sloop went to the barnyard and pulled some hair from a horse's tail. He sterilized it in boiling water and repaired the boy's face with fine horsehair sutures.

The boy was to come to the doctor's office to have the stitches removed, but he failed to appear. When he was clearly overdue, the doctor sent word to the farm that unless the sutures were removed promptly they might very well cause a horse's tail to grow from the boy's forehead. The young man appeared promptly.

Decisiveness, that is, the quick thinking required of a surgeon is not something that can be conveyed to non-surgeons, but one can gain a sense of the reflex ingenuity of accomplished surgeons from accounts of their adroitness in resolving problems outside of the operating room. In the early days of the Mayo Clinic the janitorial operations were overseen by a capable man named Jay Neville. He was highly regarded by the Mayo families, and by virtue of his long association with them addressed the doctors by their first names. Jay Neville called from the clinic one evening when Dr. Charles Mayo was at dinner.

"Charlie," he said, "You left a woman in your examining room with a speculum in her. What shall I do?"

The Mayo Clinic had become very busy, vaginal examinations for cancer were conducted on four or five women at a time. Nurses positioned the patients on examining tables in private cubicles — on their backs with legs raised and spread — and inserted a speculum, a two-bladed metal spoon in the vagina to allow the doctor to make a quick inspection for any abnormality. The doctor was supposed to follow close behind the nurse and dismiss the patient after his examination. Somehow Dr. Mayo had missed one cubicle.

Dr. Mayo resolved the dilemma immediately: "Jay," he said. "Put on a white coat, go in and take it out and tell her to return in the morning so we can continue the treatment."

At the Ochsner Clinic in New Orleans, surgeon Mims Gage, dressed in his street clothes, paused at the nurses station and was told that an elderly woman was due in the operating room, but refused to go until she had seen a Methodist minister. No minister was available. She was not his patient, but Dr. Gage offered to help. He walked into the patient's room, said he was a retired Methodist bishop, and that he would be pleased to help. He took her hand and prayed earnestly. She thanked him when he finished, relaxed, and went calmly to the operating room.

When she was recovering, walking in the corridors, she spotted Dr. Gage in a surgeon's gown and upbraided him as an impostor. Gage was unruffled. "Dear lady," he said. "I am sworn to help the suffering and my prayer was as sincere as any bishop's." She laughed and was won over. "You're right," she said. "And I thank you — bishop."

Dealing with misconceptions about surgery is harder. Ophthalmologist Edward Gifford operated on a man for a crossed eye. The result was satisfactory and the patient was pleased, but he told Dr. Gifford that the doctor might be interested to know that he had replaced the eye upside down. The patient obviously believed that an ocular surgeon can remove an eye from its socket and replace it in the course of an operation (this cannot be done). He thought he had discovered that a small mark formerly in the lower part of the eye was now in the upper part of the eye. Dr. Gifford wrote, "I tried to correct the misconception but 1 suspect he thought me a poor sport who would not admit a minor error."

The number of patient misconceptions surrounding surgery is almost infinite, and the associated emotions are often volatile. Dr. George King devised a Human Nature Chart, a basic guide for surgeons through the turbulent psychic atmosphere that surrounds every operation. The normal line of gratitude is graphed at zero on the chart. Senior surgeons counsel their students never to expect gratitude. Important fluctuations of patient attitude are indicated above and below this line beginning with the day of entry to the hospital (point A) until well after the operation (point U). The financial highlights are starred for easy reference.

To further convey the tenets of the art, surgeons have created a marvelous fund of aphorisms. Most of them are appropriately professional: "Learning surgery is difficult, teaching it is impossible." And: "It takes ten years to learn when to operate and twenty years to learn when not to." But in a lighter vein surgeons are admonished to acquire a capacity for "masterly inactivity," that is, for calculated temporizing when a situation is in doubt. And humor leavens the wisdom: "Beware of the surgeon who is great at getting out of trouble," and "Never say oops in the operating room."

The practice of surgery is a very challenging and gratifying life. But when the memoirs are written it is not the drama of the operating room that comes center stage. Rather, it is the

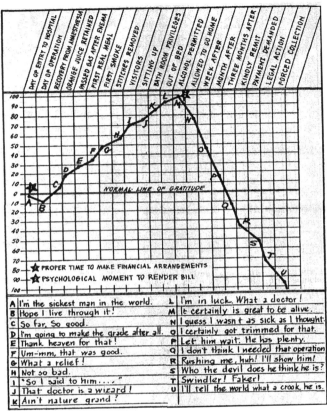

★ PROPER TIME TO MAKE FINANCIAL ARRANGEMENTS
★ PSYCHOLOGICAL MOMENT TO RENDER BILL

A	I'm the sickest man in the world.	L	I'm in luck. What a doctor!
B	Hope I live through it!	M	It certainly is great to be alive.
C	So far, So good.	N	I guess I wasn't as sick as I thought.
D	I'm going to make the grade after all.	O	I certainly got trimmed for that.
E	Thank heaven for that!	P	Let him wait. He has plenty.
F	Um-mm, that was good.	Q	I don't think I needed that operation.
G	What a relief!	R	Rushing me, huh! I'll show him!
H	Not so bad.	S	Who the devil does he think he is?
I	"So I said to him...."	T	Swindler! Faker!
J	That doctor is a wizard!	U	I'll tell the world what a crook he is.
K	Ain't nature grand?		

Human Nature Chart

small matters that revealed the best of humanity and served to recharge a surgeon's spirit over a long period when they were recalled and related. Surgeon Theron Clagett encountered a woman who needed her gall bladder removed. He discussed the operation with the patient and her husband and arranged to do it on the following day. Later in the day the doctor got a call from the woman. She had false teeth, she said, but her husband didn't know it. She knew they must come out for surgery, but would Dr. Clagett please see that they were replaced before she was returned to her room so that her husband would not discover it? Of course. Shortly thereafter, Dr. Clagett received another call. The husband called to say that his wife had false teeth, but she didn't know that he knew she had false teeth. Would Dr. Clagett kindly see that her teeth were replaced before she was returned to her room where he would meet her?

"I don't want her to know that I know," he said.

13.
Communication

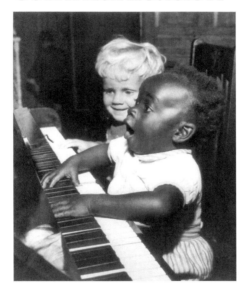

Illness evokes some striking similes and metaphors when those who are sick describe their symptoms. One who is afflicted can sometimes create in a sentence the same image that requires a paragraph in a medical textbook. A woman suffering with a bladder infection described emptying her bladder with this arresting phrase: "It feels as though I'm giving birth to a flaming lobster."

A woman suffering recurrent vertigo due to a middle-ear disturbance described the ineffable dizziness of an attack that felled her: " I felt I'd fallen off the floor and had to hang on to the carpet."

Parkinson's disease commonly causes a frozen, immobile

face with unblinking eyes and slow, deliberate movements of the limbs. A man who developed Parkinson's disease said: "I have become a lizard."

A few suffering persons have described their distress in rhyme:

> *You blush at mention of a pile.*
> *And would perhaps, the theme avoid*
> *Well, then suppose, to put on style*
> *We call the thing a hemorrhoid.*
> *You ask me by what obvious sign*
> *One may with certainty detect them*
> *Well, I can only say that mine*
> *Are like a hornet in the rectum.*

When a centenarian was asked what it felt like to be one hundred years old, he replied that it felt "like running out of gas knowing that there is no station ahead."

Those who are ill are quick to adopt the medical terms that describe their maladies and convey them to the next doctor they encounter. It is well that they do, but in the process they make some amusing transmogrifications that cause their doctors to pause. A doctor might learn that his patient had been told that he had "very close veins," and guess that the reference was to varicose veins. But it might require a thoughtful moment and a few additional questions to ascertain that the patient who spoke of "all sorts of colitis," had been told that he had ulcerative colitis. And it would be an intuitive feat for the doctor to comprehend on first-hearing that a man who was "turned down by the draft board because of corruption" was disclosing that he had a rupture or a hernia.

A malaprop oft repeated is difficult to relinquish. In the early 1980s a woman entered an inner-city Chicago emergency room and said that she was suffering from "fireballs of the Eucharist." She dismissed a medical student as "no doctor," when he said he had never heard of it. And she indignantly rejected the resident doctor because he laughed and said there was no such thing. A patient supervisory physician finally determined that the symptoms suggested fibroid of the uterus — a fairly common female affliction and that proved to be what she had. When the correct designation, fibroid of the uterus, was offered to her — for her information — she replied, "That's what I said!"

The patient who described her ailment as "roaches of the liver" surely caused her doctor a moment of consternation before cirrhosis of the liver came to mind as the proper interpretation. And the doctor could be excused for smiling when a girl with a vaginal discharge explained that she had a discharge from her "Virginia."

Tact and consideration would dictate the suppression of any sign of amusement when an elderly lady who was concerned about Alzheimer's disease asked if it was possible that she had "Old-timer's disease." But it is likely that the doctor would relate the encounter with great pleasure to the next physician he met. In turn he might be told about another lady who wondered if her difficulty remembering things might be due to the "mental pause."

Common sense leads the laity into other linguistic levity. When a resident told a contentious old fellow that his trouble was in his middle ear, the response was, "Don't be smart! I've got two like everybody else. There ain't no middle one." And similarly, a woman who was told that her painful, arthritic leg was due to old age responded that obviously age had nothing to do with it. The other leg was the same age and it was perfectly sound and supple.

When patients respond to questions in writing, the medical vocabulary is muddled in new dimensions. Dr. John Dirckx collected some examples. Describing their operations, patients told of ado (abdominal) surgery, of api ndex (appendix) operation, of removal of wisdom (teeth), and of "tubes being tide." They referred to the blatter, the glawell bladder (gall bladder), the llgu blatter, and to lymfloyd (lymphoid) glands. One described a bleeding collen (colon) and another a broken color bone.

Needless to say, medical students and residents sometimes write at similar levels of excellence. Dr. Corey Fox collected a few examples from the medical records of a general hospital in a large metropolitan area. One note read: "This mother of a two-year-old child desires a circumcision." Another note recorded that "this patient states he urinates around the clock every two hours." And one hospital record related that a "patient's wife hit him over the head with an ironing board which now has six stitches in it."

Such lapses are easy to interpret, but "geezers" create surpassing communication problems for doctors. Geezers are a special group of people distinguished in part for their ability to answer questions without conveying information. They annoy doctors, but in the end their amiability and sincerity usually win the day. Geezer is not a medical designation and the term has wide public recognition. The *New York Times,* a short time ago, carried a feature piece about two self-described geezers in Spokane, Washington. They were the proud co-owners of a Spokane deli which they had forthrightly named the "Two Geezers' Deli." Geezers are elderly, therefore the geezer element of our population is rising. Responding to this trend, the *Journal of the American Medical Association* published an article in 1988 titled, "The Assessment and Treatment of Geezers." The presentation is sober and instructive, but there is no way to suppress the comedy involved in relationships with geezers.

Doctors were counseled to avoid such introductory questions as "What brought you here?" The answer is likely to be, "A 1994 pickup truck." The question, "What do you chiefly complain of?" might be answered — after a moment of thought — by, "My wife." And if there is a hint of a urinary problem and a doctor asks, "Does your urine burn?" A geezer might well respond, "I don't know, I never tried to light it." Geezers are not a new species. Research has shown that there are "geezeresses" as well as geezers and that they were recognized and described at least as far back as 1900.

At that time an Irish geezeress in a Boston hospital was asked her age by a resident doctor and responded that she was ten years older than her sister. And her sister, she thought, was a year older than her brother. The resident wisely abandoned the subject and asked how long she had been sick. He learned that her distress — whatever it was — began about two years after her mother died. And "When?" (the imperative follow-up question), revealed that mother had never been well after father died. And of course, father died after having been ill for several years. The frustrated resident doctor made a simple last sally: "What is your trouble?" In response she asked if he was a doctor, and, upon being told that he was, she reminded him that it was his job to find out, and that it was the very thing she wanted to discover.

Geezers come in many shades. One variant was exemplified by a little old lady brought into an emergency room because she was uncommunicative and seemingly in a stuporous state. Her name and address were available from the ambulance crew, but the admitting nurse needed more information and in a face-to-face close-up she shouted, "What is your religion?"

The old woman's eyes snapped open immediately. "Why?" she asked. "Am I going to die?" "No, no, you're not going to die," the nurse reassured her. "Then I'm an atheist," the little lady sighed and subsided again into complete unresponsiveness.

But encounters with geezers are not always frustrating. Geezers have a healthy disdain for frailties and a marvelous appreciation of minor pleasures. One elderly independent geezeress when queried about food that disagreed with her, responded that, "If anything disagrees with me, I eat it until it agrees." And a man who related a progressive decline and limitation of his physical abilities added, "But I still wind the clock every Sunday morning."

Doctor-patient communication is also impeded by medical idioms that have endured in various regions of the country for generations. A graduate of a medical school in Minnesota or Iowa who became a resident in a Richmond or Atlanta hospital would be puzzled and then amused when a patient complained of "locked bowels." Southerners use the term to describe a prolonged period of bowel inaction. In some regions of the country diarrhea is described as "boweling off." To vomit may be described as to "chunk up," or to "cascade." And an infant who brought up some curdled milk might be said to have "cheesed."

One might expect that such regional idioms are rarely used, comical oddities of no practical significance. But words classed as archaic or obsolete in dictionaries are still in wide use in many regions of the United States. In 1990, investigators at the College of Medicine of the East Carolina State University published a medical lexicon for doctors and nurses in East Tennessee and adjacent Virginia and North Carolina. Studies had revealed that patients in this area couched their medical descriptions in idiomatic terms and that the doctors and nurses often failed to comprehend them. This was found to be true to an extent that sometimes caused a patient's medical needs to go unmet. The lexicon was created to improve communication and to thereby improve medical care.

The lexicon informed doctors that when a patient said he had had "a drawing spell," he had been short of breath. If he had "creeled" his ankle, he had sprained it. "Kernels" are swollen lymph glands, "knots" or "pones" are lumps under the skin, and "beals" are sore, festering lumps. If one became a boil, it was a "risen." A hemorrhoid might be called a "blood wart." "Old Arthur" is arthritis, "rigors" are chills, "janders" means jaundice, and "the whites " is a vaginal discharge. "Jack bumps" designates acne and phlebitis is called "milk leg" by many.

The genitals are "down there" or the area may be called the "privates" or the "possible." The latter term seems to have derived from nurses who when they gave bed baths told their patients that they would wash "as far up as possible and then as far down as possible." "Possible" came to define the zone where one washed oneself. A medical professional who was not a native of the region would indeed need the lexicon to function efficiently.

This difficulty of communication between doctors and their patients due to regional idioms is by no means limited to Appalachia. Dr. John Burnum described it in western Alabama in 1984. Patients told him that their feet were "strutted," when they were tight and swollen. Muscles were described as "corded," when they were stiff and painful. When they wanted something for pain, patients asked for some "nulling medicine." And if a stomach was "stubborn," the patient was constipated; if it was "torn up," diarrhea was the problem. Of course the doctor also had to command a knowledge of non-regional slang terms such as "riding the cotton pony" or "rag time" for menstruation.

When medical information is exchanged between doctors, another vocabulary appears and new words are added apace. Thus, medical jargon is created. Most of it is created by the students and the doctors in training. The medical experience is new to them, and they select fresh words to describe it. Their expressions reflect the general irreverence of younger generations, and also the stress that medical trainees have been subjected to increasingly during the last half century. By adding low-key, humorous overtones to their work, the doctors-in-training reduce tension and strengthen camaraderie.

The hospital is the jargon mill. Patients admitted to the hospital during the night and integrated into the next morning's routines are "new players." One who is admitted for treatment that may improve his condition but will not cure it, is in for a "tune-up." If it has been determined in the emergency room that the patient is indigent, it might be noted that "a negative wallet biopsy" has been done.

Moving a patient to another section of the hospital may

be referred to as "turfing" him. It is often appropriate for more efficient care, but occasionally it represents a resident doctor's effort to rid himself of a difficult patient, and the receiving resident may raise objections and defend his turf if he senses that the transfer is a ploy. "Buffing the chart" refers to updating and filling in, in anticipation of transfer of a patient or inspection by superiors.

A patient who is a diagnostic enigma might be referred to as having "GOK's disease:" God Only Knows.

One who is desperately ill might lead a resident to refer the situation as one calling for "resurrectine," a fantasy drug, sometimes called the "Jesus drug," the only thing that could possibly be helpful. A patient whose condition has deteriorated suddenly has "crumped" or "crashed." And if his condition continues grave he might be referred to as "circling the drain" or "on the launching pad" or "epitaph bound."

If his condition is hopeless, he is "booked."

If the oscillations traced on the electrocardiogram subside to a flat line — indicating failed heart function — it is the "Nebraska sign," and signals a demise. Some call it the "Holland sign." A patient who died has "boxed" or "escaped into space" or "gone to glory."

There are doubtless more euphemisms for death and burial than for any other human state. The polite ones are well known; the slang phrases are risible; a few of each are listed below:

> *Grounded for good*
> *Gone aloft*
> *Now installed in furnace No. 10*
> *Put to bed with a shovel*
> *Gone to grass*
> *In the ETU (eternal care unit, the morgue)*
> *Called "Out" by the big umpire*
> *Transferred to Big Sky General*
> *Transferred to ward X*

Planted

A postmortem pathology conference for the trainee staff may be referred to as the "man-in-the-pan conference," the organs of interest being on view and available for inspection in a large laboratory pan. Attending doctors sometimes refer to the conference as an "organ recital." The organs come from the "Temple of Truth" — the morgue.

On a surgical floor, the "lipstick sign" is important. It means that a female patient is sufficiently improved to have resumed applying her lipstick — a very good sign.

A resident doctor who found it difficult to say rectum and vagina to his female patients adopted the terms "back passage" and "front passage" instead. A patient validated his choices by adding another expression to the genre. She called on the telephone to report that she was bleeding "from below." When asked "from where below," she replied: "From the gentleman's passage."

In the emergency room there are "GOMERS." The word is an acronym for Get Out of My Emergency Room. Amiable residents read it as Grand Old Men of the Emergency Room — most GOMERS are men. It applies to persons who haunt emergency rooms for various behavioral reasons: those who appear repeatedly because of alcoholism and drug abuse, some who arrive with self-inflicted injuries and some with self-induced physiological changes, all seeking a few free meals and a clean bed. There is a group who are tormented by health fears. They appear repeatedly with baseless complaints and refuse to accept reassurance. They want tests. And there are some who feign illness for indeterminate reasons. These people consume time and resources that are in short supply and would be better devoted to others. They are not medical emergencies — they are GOMERS.

The emergency room familiarizes physicians with the argot of the narcotic addiction spectacle.

Cocaine is variously referred to as "Dr. White" (said to be

the only doctor who can be of real assistance), "snow," "happy dust," or "Charlie." Heroin may be "witch hazel." Marijuana is "Mary," "Mary Jane," "grass," "hay," or "locoweed." Narcotics generally are "junk," and barbiturates are "goofballs."

Some addicts will "do a Brodie" (a bizarre, seizure-like contortion or gyration, named for Steve Brodie who jumped off the Brooklyn Bridge to call attention to himself). These exhibitions are also called "twisters" or "cartwheels" and are intended to invite injections of sedative drugs. Another addict may be in are a genuine "panic," a delirium similar to that seen with alcohol. Hypodermic needles are "guns," "harpoons," or "artillery." A syringe may be a "pistol" and veins are referred to as "up and down lines."

The medical jargon includes a collection of euphemisms that designate patient categories. The euphemisms permit medical discussions when they might otherwise have to be abandoned for fear that clear and forthright words would be regarded as offensive by a patient, relatives, or even other doctors. Many of these euphemisms are of literary derivation. Dr. Osler at Johns Hopkins was a great exponent of them. For Osler a drunkard was a "disciple of Bacchus." A patient with venereal disease was a "devotee of Eros," or a "client of Venus." His affliction might be spoken of as "aphroditis."

Emergency room communication is facilitated if the medical staff is versed in euphemisms for drunkenness. Benjamin Franklin compiled and published a list of more than two hundred in 1737; some are still useful — and diverting:

Been in the sun
Lordly
Got on his little hat
He's a king
Cherubinical
In his prosperity
Top heavy
He sees two moons

A ready bank of euphemisms for mental disturbances also promotes medical communication in the emergency room. Dr Thomas Sasz compiled a helpful lexicon. A disturbed person may be: A Bedlamite, in the ozone, a few quarts low, shrink bait, fifty cents on the dollar, up the flue foo foo, out to lunch.

This working jargon it does not appear on hospital records. There is an additional "medicalese" composed of metaphors, acronyms, eponyms and abbreviations that is used extensively in hospital records. Laity who review medical records — librarians, insurance examiners and government analysts — are likely to be puzzled by some words and frustrated by abbreviations.

A medical librarian at Duke University was offended when she repeatedly encountered the abbreviation S.O.B. on the charts of patients being treated at the university hospital. She sent a memo to Dr. Eugene Stead, the professor of medicine indicating that she found the abbreviation distasteful and that it would surely reflect on the university if it was encountered by outsiders. She suggested that Dr. Stead institute a campaign to eliminate it.

Dr. Stead replied that "the abbreviation S.O.B., for shortness of breath, is in nationwide use and we will be unable to stop its appearing in Duke records."

The longest abbreviation is also in widespread use; it is a great time-saver: "WDWNWM-NAD," which stands for, a "well-developed, well-nourished, white male, in no acute distress," is easily varied to cover a female or an African American. "TLC," for tender, loving care, has spread far beyond the hospitals. And there is a well known humorous abbreviation that is probably fictitious: "3-H enema," an abbreviated directive for a nurse to administer an enema high, hot, and a hell of a lot.

Abbreviations can mislead — even be dangerous. There is "TAB," meant to stand for triple antibiotic. In one instance when a doctor ordered irrigation with a TAB solution, it caused a wound to be irrigated with a popular diet soda.

Recording their examinations, doctors write metaphorically of horseshoe kidneys, strawberry tongues, pigeon chests and butterfly (shaped) rashes. Nurses give patients sponge "doughnuts" to protect their heels from pressure, bring them "soft trays" to eat from, tell them when they can "dangle" and apply "butterflies" (tapes), to hold infusion needles in place on the skin.

Medicine has its acronyms to convey information economically. "CABG" is one. It stands for coronary artery bypass graft — a heart operation. If verbalized, the operation is a "cabbage" operation, and the patient who has undergone one has been "cabbaged."

Eponyms play a large role in both the speech and writings of doctors. Physicians' names are attached to diseases they have defined. Sometimes a disease is named for a mythical or literary character. There is Addison's disease, named for Dr. Thomas Addison who recognized it; the Pickwick syndrome, named for the fat boy described by Charles Dickens in the *Pickwick Papers;* and an Alice in Wonderland syndrome in which the size, shape and position of things is disordered — usually after a stroke.

The Lazarus syndrome is a modern addition. It applies to some persons who have suffered a cardiac arrest and have been resuscitated. As far as we know Lazarus was none the worse for having been revived, but modern resuscitated persons often suffer mental difficulties.

The resuscitation experience has produced interesting observations on the hereafter. One resuscitated person had his atheistic beliefs confirmed. Of his adventure to the Great Perhaps, he said, "There is nothing there." But another such person had his faith vindicated. He said, "There seemed to be music and angels singing on the other side." Many who have been rescued from death have nothing to report. The happening is now called the Near Death Experience. Reports of it are accumulating at a furious pace, but enlightenment derived from them, so far, has been nil.

The sufferings of the saints covers a substantial part of the disease spectrum. Doctors with clerical or antiquarian tastes can spice their work with saintly references. There is St. Anthony's Fire, used by some to designate shingles and by others to identify erysipelas; both conditions are characterized by areas of fiery red skin. If you have a toothache you are suffering St. Apollonia's syndrome.

St. Fiacre suffered so mightily from hemorrhoids that his name was attached to the disorder. St. Martin's syndrome reminds us that alcoholism even invaded the ranks of the saints, and if you have contracted St. Sebastian's syndrome, you have acquired plague. There are more than thirty diseases associated with the names of the saints.

The Ulysses syndrome describes a circuitous voyage often taken by a physician and his patient in the course of a medical investigation. It is initiated when a laboratory test is reported to be abnormal — by mistake. A multitude of factors prevent a physician from ignoring the test result — even if his judgment tells him to do so — and of course the patient usually wants it pursued. So additional tests are undertaken to pursue the false lead of the mistaken test, which results in a great circle of examinations and tests — both physically and financially trying as they are suffered through — leading back to the point of departure as in Ulysses' ten-year odyssey.

Some afflictions are identified by names that have amusing connotations. There is Saturday Night Palsy, a common paralysis of the wrist muscles of one arm. It usually strikes Saturday night drinkers and implies not making it into bed because of inebriation. Typically the subject has fallen asleep in an armchair and slept so soundly with one arm pressed against the unyielding arm of the chair that nerve damage occurs and he awakens with a paralyzed arm. A principal arm nerve is close to the surface and vulnerable to pressure just where an arm would commonly rest under the weight of one's body against a chair's armrest.

The Chinese Restaurant syndrome has been quite widely publicized, It occur about twenty minutes after the meal. It features burning sensations in the neck, arms and chest with some chest pain. It raises fears of a heart attack, but it represents a sensitivity to monosodium glutamate, which is much used in Chinese cooking.

Nurses share the medical vocabulary with the doctors and supplement it with a jargon of their own suited to their special tasks. They give "meds" (medications), take "vitals "(temperature, pulse etc.), dispense "monkey jackets" (hospital gowns), and inquire about "BMs." The male urinal is a duck or a vase and the bedpan may be either a bucket or a throne.

Nurses may refer to the "ICU" (intensive care unit) as the rose room because of the fragility of the patients under treatment there or in stressful periods refer to it as the pressure cooker. If a patient "arrests" (has heart stoppage), the nurse calls for a "crash cart"(a miniature rescue van) and may "pump the patient" (initiate heart massage by repetitive chest compression) or "bag the patient" (pump oxygen into the lungs from a handheld apparatus).

In the operating room the "scrub" nurse (sterile and assisting the surgeon) and a "dirty" nurse more politely referred to as the circulating nurse (a non-sterile assistant) are distinct. Both are designated modified angels. The anesthetist is the "gas-passer" and the laboratory technicians are "vampires." Hospital ambulances are variously designated trauma trucks, meat wagons or agony wagons and, sometimes more genteelly, as hospital limousines. To lighten the somber aura generally attached to these vehicles, hospital attendants like to tell of the Mrs. Malaprop who informed them that she came to the hospital in an "avalanche."

The most important medical communication is that which passes the gleanings of experience from skilled physicians to their juniors. Most of it cannot be put into words. It can only be learned by observation and emulation, but aphorisms can provide some memorable summaries. The ancients cautioned their students that "doctors treat, but nature cures." This great insight was updated recently by a Boston physician who told his students repeatedly: "Don't get in nature's way." It has been noted that "masterly inactivity" is sometimes the best course for a wise surgeon to follow. A similar counsel applies to physicians generally. The best care is sometimes "audacious inaction."

There are aphorisms that transmit useful medical information to the public. Oliver Wendell Holmes offered a facetious prescription for a long life: "The best way to live long is to get a chronic disease and take good care of it." Dr. Charles Earle offered a caution that should be added to all advisories on how to pick a doctor: "The best doctors sign the most death certificates." In the popular vein there is: "Never use a doctor whose office plants are dying."

Despite considerable experience with the problems of communication, medical writers require the critical cooperation of medical editors when they want transmit ideas with insured clarity and concision. Geniality governs success. Dr. Eugene Stead had a manuscript returned by an editor and found the editing not to his liking. Dr. Stead's personality featured a straightaway attitude that colored his actions, speech and writing. He wrote a note to the editor: "I appreciate the time and thought you spent in editing my manuscript.... I have a style of speaking and writing which is well known to a number of generations of students at many levels. I would prefer to keep my somewhat idiomatic approach rather than use your changes, which in terms of projecting anyone but myself are obvious improvements."

Dr. Charles Mayo once completed a medical manuscript and sent it to Maude Mellish, the clinic's internal editor for staff publications. After an interval the manuscript came back across Dr. Mayo's busy desk and he read it. Then he penned a note to Mellish. "Interesting paper," he said, "Who wrote it?"

14.
Laughter
in the Library

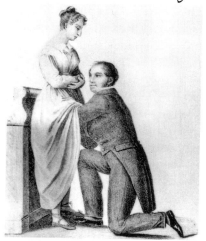

Obstetrical examination

When professional medical journals publish studies that are subject to alternative conclusions, or pieces with pompous or careless assertions, doctors are quick to write critical corrective letters to the editors, and sometimes to offer witty, dissenting interpretations.

In 1985 the *Journal of the American Medical Association* published a study of the medical needs of the homeless. A survey had found that among the homeless, 10 percent had high blood pressure, 5 percent suffered from arthritis, and 2 percent were diabetic. The figures were said to demonstrate that the homeless had unmet medical needs.

A physician reader wrote to the editor to say that in his office, among his patients, the figures were much higher: 30 percent had high blood pressure, 25 percent had arthritis, and 20 percent were diabetic. It was clear, he wrote, that the difference in the two sets of figures allowed an additional conclusion and that he was acting on it. He was now advising his patients to take to the road — homelessness appeared to be good for your health.

In addition to commenting on published studies, doctors write in to report untoward effects of new drugs and new procedures. It is important that such information be disseminated promptly. Among the new heart tests, one involves the injection of radioactive thallium. The thallium remains in the body for several days after the test and is slowly eliminated. Some bank vaults have radiation detectors to detect and prevent the placement of any radioactive substances in the vault boxes.

A patient who had a thallium heart test went to his bank's safety deposit vault on the following day and set off the bank's alarm system. His doctor wrote to the editor of a widely read medical journal warning that a thallium heart test could freeze a patient's assets for more than a week.

Magnetic resonance imaging (MRI) was also found to pose a potential financial complication — this one for physicians. In the course of an MRI scan a patient exhibited some distress and a doctor stuck his head and shoulders into the machine to assist the patient. The physician had his wallet in the shirt pocket of his hospital garb. A few days later the doctor entered his card at an ATM and it was repeatedly rejected. Then he visited a restaurant and his Visa and American Express cards were both rejected. All of the cards in his wallet had been demagnetized by the scanner.

When new medical techniques are introduced, they are likely to be modified and improved almost immediately since letters to the editors of the professional journals keep the profession up to date. Cardiopulmonary resuscitation — CPR — has been much publicized and widely adopted by the public as a first aid measure. A letter to the editor of a principal medical journal described a modification of the standard CPR technique encountered by the physician-writer. The published letter was captioned: "CPR: The P Stands for Plumber's Helper." It told of a man with known heart disease who collapsed and did not respond to his son's attempt to administer CPR. The son knew about CPR, but was unpracticed in the technique. When it failed, he ran for the toilet plunger and applied it vigorously to his father's chest — and the stricken man came to life.

At the hospital, the euphoric son recommended that a plumber's plunger be placed at the side of each bed in the cardiac care unit. The doctors recommended that he take a basic CPR course and learn how to do it right, but they admitted that it was hard to argue with success.

The story has a comical sequel. Four years later, in the same medical journal, the doctor who had related this incident described a new device for CPR. It had a suction cup like a plumber's plunger with a doorknob-like handle for easy application of pressure. It was to be applied to the chest and "plunged," and in some cases it worked better than standard CPR.

A technique such as CPR, in the hands of laymen, is certain to be sometimes misapplied. Fortunately, misapplication is usually harmless — but it can be trying for the subject. A letter to the editor told of a man afflicted with Menier's disease — recurrent episodes of prostrating dizziness due to inner ear malfunction — who was felled in a public place. He was too dizzy to move a muscle. Well-intentioned laymen straddled him immediately and gave him CPR enthusiastically, though it was utterly inappropriate. The poor fellow was helpless while his lungs were blown into and his chest squeezed and he described it as the worst experience of his entire life.

But it could have been worse. A man who collapsed at a social function was revived by a bartender who had been trained in CPR. The ill man was then hospitalized by ambulance and support of his heart saved his life. But on the sixth hospital day he developed a fever, hoarseness, and difficulty breathing. An x-ray showed a partial dental plate lodged in his lower throat. It belonged to the bartender who had lost it during mouth to mouth resuscitation.

A great number of people have been instructed in CPR as a first aid measure. Now anyone who loses consciousness is likely to be subjected to it. This has defined a group of people, some of whom for one reason or another do not want to be resuscitated and some of whom fear that for some reason CPR might be applied to them by mistake. How to make one's wish known in a way that will prevail? In an attempt to solve this dilemma a few persons have had "Do Not Resuscitate" or "No CPR" tattooed across the front of their chest.

Good Samaritans are blithely unaware of the diagnostic traps that surround them when they sally to a rescue. Dr. Edith Johnson told of being in church in Palo Alto, California, when a woman sitting across the aisle and in front of her began to attract some attention. Her head fell back suddenly and her mouth hung open. The equivalent of a death rattle came forth from her throat. The minister noticed and looked startled. The scene was alarming and a good Christian sitting behind the lapsing lady was incited to intervene.

He moved out into the aisle and then to the side of the afflicted woman — something had to be done. He scooped her up in his arms and started to carry her out of the church, when she suddenly came to life. She had fallen asleep — and she was very upset. Her would-be rescuer put her down and sat beside her for a moment while the congregation tried to smother its laughter. The woman cast repetitive hateful looks at the crestfallen man and, after a few minutes and rising embarrassment, drove him out of the church.

Though it seems rather unlikely, it is clear that some reactions to medical therapy are reactions to the treatment and the doctor. A cancer specialist wrote to the editor of the *New England Journal of Medicine* calling attention to this previously unreported phenomenon. He told of treating a woman with cancer, by chemotherapy. Chemotherapy often provokes nausea and vomiting during the course of treatment and that was the case in this instance. Several weeks after the woman had been treated, the doctor chanced to encounter her in a shopping mall. At the first sight of him, she immediately threw up.

Editors have great opportunities to lighten the generally sober pages of their publications by permitting or devising arresting titles for their published pieces and we are indebted to those who do. The *New England Journal* caught its readers' eyes and elevated their spirits when it published a report titled "Mediastinal Emphysema After a Sax Orgy." Mediastinal emphysema designates the presence of air in the tissues surrounding the heart. It is abnormal and it is a threat to heart function. In this instance it was caused by a tiny rupture of the lung during a spell of vigorous saxophone playing associated with expressive body contortions and gyrations. The combined blowing and gyrating so increased the pressure in the lungs that an internal blowout occurred. Fortunately, the musician made an uncomplicated recovery. His doctors advised him to practice safe sax in the future.

The same journal once ran an editorial about the relief of itching which was titled: "Itching Research Has Barely Scratched the Surface." And the *New York State Medical Journal* published a piece about a man who had a cardiac transplant titled: "He Had a Change of Heart."

But editors must be careful in their choice of subjects when they dispense humor. A humorous article on chicken soup was preceded by an editorial that made sure the readers would recognize it as humorous. For some, chicken soup is a serious subject. Maimonides, in the 12th century, thought it had great medicinal value and it has been alleged that the recipe was given to Moses on Mount Sinai. Its prestige endures.

When a new disease is recognized and described, careful consideration must be given to naming it. The name must have elasticity in order to accommodate additional manifestations of the disease which are certain to be found by others as more is learned about it. In 1956 neurologists at the Mayo Clinic recognized a new disease characterized by remarkable muscle stiffness. They studied it, published a report describing it, and called it, "The Stiff Man Syndrome."

Perhaps the name was as great a stimulus as the report itself for the worldwide search that followed for additional cases of this new disease. If so, British physicians soon found what they were looking for. Two years after the Mayo report, British doctors published an article titled "A Woman With the Stiff Man Syndrome." And subsequently, the same condition was found in a child.

Other new diseases, "diseases of progress," are appearing at an alarming rate. They are named as they are encountered and doctors are alerted to watch for them "Pizza Palsy" is a newly recognized disability. It is a partial paralysis of a hand incurred by commercial pizza cutters. The repetitive pressure of the roller-blade injures a vulnerable nerve at the base of the little finger.

Another more extensive hand paralysis called "Vegas Neuropathy" seems to be increasing rapidly.

It is caused by prolonged leaning on an elbow at a gaming table. It was first reported in Las Vegas, Nevada, but it has also been reported in Atlantic City and has cropped up on Indian reservations and along the Mississippi River.

The "Backyard Barbecue Syndrome" is now a securely established medical entity and is a medical emergency. Steaks cooked in the back yard are commonly overdone— firm, crusted and difficult to chew up adequately. The elderly are particularly prone to swallow a piece that only goes halfway down where it lodges to obstruct the esophagus. A prompt hospital visit is then required.

As more people acquire dogs for protection, the incidence of "Dog Walker's Elbow" is increasing steadily. This painful affliction develops when an elbow joint is repetitively tugged on at awkward angles as the dog on the end of the leash searches the bushes and trash containers, chases cats and sniffs fireplugs.

Euthanasia is one thing, but head-in-the-clouds philosophers have debated seriously for the past twenty years whether or not the elderly and disabled have a separate and distinct duty to die. Is it their duty to their family to relieve them of the burden of care and their duty to the world's poor to free up resources for their benefit? Could be a whole new arena of medical action — but it is destined to crash.

Some old diseases are given new modes of transmission by new inventions and require new measures to control their menace. Gonorrhea is generally referred to in medicalese as "GC." It is sexually transmitted and its control is dependent upon finding the infected persons and treating them. This a public health task undertaken by our public health doctors and nurses.

As chatting over the CB radio waves became increasingly popular many new social networks developed including one that offered female companionship to CB'er truck drivers. One result was a plague of GC, referred to in this instance as "CBGC" by public health officials because it was a special variety: one in which they were unable to find the sources of the infection and treat them. Doctors urged the CB'ers to make the infected parties known among themselves — over the airwaves. In this way, doctors said, the drivers could avoid the plague effectively with less effort and ingenuity than they already devoted to avoiding "Smokey." This network has now moved to the Internet, with an increased risk of contracting and spreading the disease.

Inasmuch as most medical literature is somber, authors are tempted to devise witty opening lines to entice readers.

A doctor who had accidentally walked through a plate glass door thought worthy of reporting that in addition to numerous lacerations, he was left with a phobic fear of all expanses of glass that caused him much anxiety and lasted for nine months. His account began: "Walking through a pane of glass is a shattering experience."

When a single line provokes laughter in the middle of a sober piece, one can never know if it is a slip of the mind or an impish indulgence by the author. A recent study on the feeding of infants, for example, includes the observation that: "Many general practitioners pay only lip service to breast feeding." And a paper affirming, on the basis of new experimental evidence, that the bladder is an active contracting and relaxing organ, not simply a passive receptacle, concluded that: "The concept of the bladder as an inert container of urine no longer holds water."

Many medical journals welcome articles about the artistic and literary manifestations of medicine; they relieve the doctors' reading. Most of them are airy speculations. One pondered the effect of Robert Louis Stevenson's tuberculosis on his writings. Another debated the correct diagnosis of the ailment that troubled painter Vincent van Gogh: was it epilepsy, middle ear disease, or brain syphilis? And one romantic described in detail how Romeo might have saved Juliet if he had been versed in CPR.

A prestigious medical journal published a piece by a professor of chemistry at a large university explaining how Lot's wife was transformed into a pillar of salt: it was a blast of hot air from the burning city that did it, and he ventured further into the ether by concluding "we see how modern science corroborates medical events described in the Bible." Two university professors of chemistry wrote in to say, "nonsense" — and a debate ensued that lasted more than a year in subsequent issues.

And there is the enigma of the thought behind Mona Lisa's smile. Some have opined that it is because she knows she is pregnant and others that it is because she knows she isn't. Doctor speculate about the marvelous painting by Luke Fildes, "The Doctor." What is he thinking? Jesters suggest that he has forgotten the dose of the drug he wants to use and is trying to think of it.

A doctor traveling in Italy viewed Michelangelo's sculpture of David and came away puzzled. The Jewish biblical hero was depicted uncircumcised. How could this be? How could Michelangelo make such a mistake? The doctor sent the question off in a letter to a medical editor.

The question went unanswered, but elicited a letter from a physician-reader that indicated a wide recognition of it and how others had reacted to it. He told of reproductions of the David in which he is circumcised and of others in which the question is disposed of with a fig leaf. One has a choice. Michelangelo created another anatomical enigma. On the ceiling of the Sistine Chapel he painted Adam with a navel. Adam was created whole. He didn't need a navel. Would God create a useless navel? Raphael also depicted Adam with a navel, and this has provoked tortuous discussions ever since.

A more practical anatomical question is: Why do men have breasts? This was debated in nineteenth century lyceums. Abraham Lincoln interested himself in discussions of this riddle.

Despite the fact that there is nothing new to be said on the subject, writings on ethics have proliferated. They commonly involve a quotation from the third century B.C. document called the Hippocratic Oath and a complaint that in the course of a recent encounter with a physician some aspect of the oath was violated. Doctors are amused. The Hippocratic Oath is a historical treasure. Its tenets are timeless. But this is the twenty-first century; the oath would need an update if it was to be relevant. Satirical imitations make the point. A recent one reads in part: "I will prescribe regimens for the good of my patients according to my ability and judgment, but never violate the rules of Medicare, Medicaid, HMOs,

PPOs (preferred provider organization) and the like. I will never keep a patient in the hospital longer than the DRG allows or the HMOs and PPOs suggest, regardless of the inconvenience to my patient. I will always use generic drugs, even if I think the proprietary version is more effective. I will always obtain a second opinion even if I do not think one is necessary and the patient does not want one. I will try to ration the resources spent on my patients in line with federal, state and insurance company mandates."

The significance of the Hippocratic Oath is the spirit, not the letter. Dr. William Osler stated it succinctly in a form that needs no update. He said: "Live the Golden Rule."

Ethicists have aroused appreciable sympathy for a moral that would oblige doctors to always tell the whole truth. It is a naive and mischievous demand. Dr. Douglas Bond, a psychiatrist at Western Reserve University, illustrated why. He told of a man who wrote a forthright essay titled "I Have Cancer," which was reprinted in the *Reader's Digest*. The author received some four hundred thousand letters from readers expressing their pleasure with the candor and valor of his account. While these responses were accumulating, the author lost more than a hundred pounds and required transfusions for survival. At this point he queried his doctor, "Doc, what are my chances?" The doctor was surprised and replied with what he assumed was the forthrightness expected and desired by the patient: "Only a miracle can save you," he said. The patient, his wife, and some friends, all promptly "became hysterical."

Long ago Oliver Wendell Holmes advised doctors that: "Your patient has no more right to know all the truth that you know than he has to all the medicine in your bag."

"How to" articles are popular in all periodicals. In medical journals they deal with the practical aspects of doctoring, and wags invade the genre for amusement.

Writing has become a burden for doctors. They write on hospital charts, office records, insurance forms and in innumerable reports to other doctors, lawyers, and government agencies. Dr. Stanley Schwartz called attention to a way of reducing the burden:

"When I was yungr, I rmembr reding signs in the NYC subway advertising a school that teaches SPDWR IT1NG. The ads claimed, "If u cn rd ths, u cn gt a gud jb." of crse I cd rd tht! Wh cldn't? Nw her 1 am a physcn prctsing mdcne (gnrlly cnsdred a gud jb), having to write dtaild prgss rites al dy lng in rgulr oldfshnd frml English ...lmgne th time savings if we al cld rd and wrte ths wy!"

Reading is also a burden. The progress of science is so swift and wide that more is being published than the doctor can read, but there is another reason.

Young doctors are anxious to become medical authors; it is the path to prestige and to academic advancement. As a result they are commonly incautious and publish observations that are soon discredited. This is a burden to readers.

Fortunately, it is now well recognized that premature publication is also a burden for an ambitious young doctor. A discredited article may be cited by other writers for years with a warning that its conclusions are erroneous. The author is careless and unreliable. One prestigious academic, burdened with such a discredited first publication, remarked ruefully that he was less fortunate than a friend of his whose first manuscript was lost in the mail and never published.

To some extent errant publications are inevitable. Theories are proven wrong and abandoned, and longer experience often reverses short-term enthusiasms. But the publications survive and continue to be read — worse, they continue to be acted upon. University of Michigan neurosurgeon Dr. Edgar Kahn proposed a solution. Dr. Kahn suggested that there be a Journal of Retractions, a journal in which published medical information later shown to be erroneous could be openly retracted. His suggestion stemmed from an unsettling personal experience.

In 1947 Dr. Kahn published the details of a new spinal operation to relieve a common variety of leg paralysis. He had devised the operation and performed it several times and he thought that the results were very good. But other neuro-surgeons found the operation to be useless and with further experience Dr. Kahn agreed he had been mistaken.

Twenty years later, Dr. Kahn visited medical clinics in Europe to observe and learn what he could from foreign neurosurgeons. On a visit to one hospital he was directed to an operating room to observe and told that the surgeon was about to do a "Kahn operation." Dr. Kahn was astonished, "Why?" he asked. "The operation is no good." It had been abandoned and it didn't work. His host listened politely and led him into an operating room where the operation was in progress. He introduced the visitor to the surgeon and, almost as an afterthought, he asked, "What did you say your name was?"

A doctor's best effort to be forthright can be countered by a patient's wish or need to believe. A Chicago neurosurgeon told how he devised an operation he hoped would relieve a congenital weakness of the legs that is common in children. He did the operation on a few children and it failed, so he gave it up. Twenty years later he encountered the mother of one of the children. "Are you still doing the operation you performed on Jack?" she asked. The surgeon said no, and when she asked why, he said, "Because it didn't do any good." Jack was one of the failures, but his mother said, "Oh, wasn't Jack lucky, he got such a good result."

Some bits of medical literature are intentionally mislead-ing, read with great confidence and pleasure and no harm done. Literary hoaxes are pure fun. Their essence is amuse-ment, no fraud or exploitation is involved. Between 1887 and 1900, *Appleton's Cyclopaedia of American Biography* was published in seven volumes. It was subsequently found to contain at least eighty-four biographies of persons who never existed, including one of a doctor who was credited with controlling a cholera epidemic that never occurred. In 1946 a medical publication of the Welsh National School of Medicine at Cardiff, Wales, lent credence to a comical hoax when it published a communication from a special correspondent in New York. The writer purported to describe a newly discovered work of Hippocrates. This ancient document included medical aphorisms never before associated with the name of Hippocrates. One aphorism was said to read: "The absence of respiration is a bad sign." Another asserted that "Hemorrhoids are not improved by horseback riding," and a third that: "Drowsiness and the itch are incompatible."

The longest running medically related hoax was written by H.L. Mencken in 1917. Mencken recounted the history of the first bathtub in America. It was displayed, he wrote, in Cincinnati in 1842. It was made of mahogany, lined with lead, and inaugurated at a stag party at which all of the guests tried it out. But bathtubs were denounced as dangerous by physicians, banned in Boston, and heavily taxed elsewhere in efforts to suppress them. This tale has been referred to and quoted from by serious historians and sociologists repeatedly right up to the present year. Mencken said it never occurred to him that anyone would take it seriously.

Wallace Rayburn published a book in 1971 relating the history of the flush toilet. The device was said to have been invented by a Thomas Crapper and the book was titled, *Flushed With Pride.* This hoax has also been given a place in some serious discussions by the unwary, last in 1996 in a biography of a surgeon.

Many contemporary physicians sense an adversarial element in their relationships with the public. Some think there is a war going on. They are correct. The longest skirmish in history is the one between doctors and their patients and no cessation of the fray is in sight. Plato complained that doctors were making the Greeks sick.

In Roman times Pliny wrote that doctors had "ruined the

morals of the Empire." Mercifully, the Dark Ages hid physicians' machinations through the next several centuries, but in the fourteenth century Erasmus found medicine to be a "compound of imposture and craft." During the Renaissance, Petrarch wrote that more people died with a doctor's care than without it. One can allow something for the needs of drama when Shakespeare wrote, "Trust not the physician," but his insights are generally regarded as those of a genius. Thomas Jefferson thought doctors were destroyers of health and in contemporary times Ralph Nader, speaking before a congressional committee, said that it was "debatable that the aggregate health of this country is being advanced by the medical profession."

Medical librarians exert themselves to keep doctors informed of what the public is reading. They often set up a conspicuous, portable shelf of current sociological books and park it at the entrance to the book stacks so that doctors will be certain to encounter it. The shelf delivers a shock to the young doctors just out of medical school because it stands much of what he has just learned on its head There are titles such as *Examining Your Doctor* and *Talk Back to Your Doctor,* and when he encounters the book titled *Managing Your Doctor,* it becomes clear that caring for a patient can become something of a tussle. Dr. Osler, a most compassionate man, acknowledged the dilemma: "It must be confessed," he wrote, "that the practice of medicine among our fellow creatures is often a testy and choleric business."

Medical practice calls for tact. Experienced doctors define and exemplify it. Dr. John DaCosta defined tact for his students in Philadelphia. He wrote: "It consists of telling a squint-eyed man that he has fine, firm chin." And Dr. Leo Davidoff set a splendid example of a tactful description and treatment of a medical colleague. Dr. Davidoff was asked if he had anything to add to a biographical sketch of a surgeon under whom he had once served as a subordinate, and who was a notably irascible and difficult man. Dr. Davidoff replied:

"I can say nothing good about that bastard and I won't say anything bad."

Dr. DaCosta served up another bit of wisdom that has wide application in medicine: Things are not always what they seem. He told of a physician friend who gained a wide reputation for dignity because he had a stiff neck and a stiff back due to rheumatism.

Medicine owes its progress to the application of science, but even in scientific medicine things are not always what they seem.

Journal editors keep the subject of scientific methods before their readers, and doctors must judge the validity of studies claiming great virtues for new drugs and new operations.

On an elementary level, for instance, they must understand the "placebo effect."

The placebo effect is the remarkable fact that any drug given for any condition to anyone produces improvement with an incidence of some 35 percent. Operations have a similar placebo effect as do doctors. The simple presence, reassurance and laying on of hands by the doctor has a placebo effect — it relieves things. It has been said that any doctor who doesn't have a placebo effect should relinquish the profession.

Scientific evaluations call for "controlled studies" to eliminate the misleading placebo effect. In a controlled study the effect of a drug being tested is compared to the result in a comparable group of patients receiving a sugar pill. Controlled studies — when they demonstrate that a drug is useless — may have the comical result of depriving both patients and doctors of the use of a drug they were perfectly happy with. They both may have thought it was good and effective. Both were misled by the placebo effect. And they don't relinquish their confidence easily. They often protest that it really did help. It is estimated that 35 to 45 percent of today's medical prescriptions are unlikely to have any specific effect on the conditions they are prescribed for.

But controlled studies have their own flaws, and they are not applicable in some types of investigations, so additional procedures and new precautions have to be devised to minimize errors and find the truth. And they in turn have flaws, and additional rules of proof must be devised. And as the structure of science is created, one comes to the discomfiting realization that science cannot prove anything. It can only disprove our conceptions of things, It can never reach the truth, but can only get closer and closer — infinitely: "All truths are half-truths."

Medicine is not science; it is an art based on science. The doctor is called upon to comprehend the structure of science, but he also must know his patient. He is called upon to allay apprehension, minimize distress, and to encourage maximum cooperation for recovery. But, alas, in this endeavor, too, the doctor must function in the absence of ever knowing the truth. Oliver Wendell Holmes recognized that the patient known to himself and the patient known to his maker are totally different than the patient known to us.

The milieu of healing teems with uncertainties. What sort of person is fitted to be a healer?

Two prayers for doctors plead for the requisite endowments. The first is earnest:

From the inability to leave well enough alone, from too much zest for what is new and contempt for what is old, from putting knowledge before wisdom, service before art, cleverness before common sense from treating patients as cases, and from making the cure of disease more grievous than its endurance, Good Lord, deliver us.

The other prayer celebrates the role of a sense of humor in a healer. It was the invocation at the meeting of the Canadian Medical Association in 1964:

Lord, Thou knowest better than I myself that I am growing older and will some day be old. Keep me from the fatal habit of thinking that I must say something on every subject and on every occasion. Release me from the craving to straighten out everybody's affairs.

Make me thoughtful, but not moody; helpful, but not bossy. With my vast store of wisdom, it seems a pity not to use it all, but Thou knowest, Lord, that I want a few friends left at the end.

Keep my mind free from the recital of endless details; give me wings to get to the point. Seal my lips on my aches and pains. They are increasing and love of rehearsing them is becoming sweeter as the years go by. I dare not ask for grace enough to enjoy the tales of others' pains, but help me to endure them with patience. I dare not ask for improved memory, but for growing humility and a lessening of cocksureness when my memory seems to clash with the memories of others. Teach me the glorious lesson that occasionally I may be mistaken.

Keep me reasonably sweet: I do not want to be a saint — some of them are hard to live with — but a sour old soul is one of the crowning works of the Devil. Give me the ability to see good things in unexpected places and unexpected talents in people and give me the grace to tell them so.

The philosophy of life embodied in these prayers must be supplemented by an attitude toward the great and final question. How do doctors see it? In 1900 Harvard University planned a series of "Lectures on Immortality." President Charles Eliot of Harvard wrote to Dr. William Welch, professor of pathology at the Johns Hopkins Medical School, and asked him to present a physician's view. Dr. Welch replied that as far he could tell science had nothing to say on the subject. Dr. Eliot wrote back that this was exactly what he wished Dr. Welch to say. But Dr. Welch replied that he could not possibly fill an hour saying so.

Philadelphia surgeon John DaCosta advised doctors not to search for final answers. He said that if the Lord came down and explained it to us we wouldn't have the capacity to understand it

Humor cushions our disquiet. Death answers the great and final question: Do we go on to something sublime?

Will the soul live free of the body? Or is death the sad end of the line?

The living won't know the answer. Perhaps it is just as well.

It would be hard to go on without heaven. And who would be good without hell?

15.
Discovery and Innovation

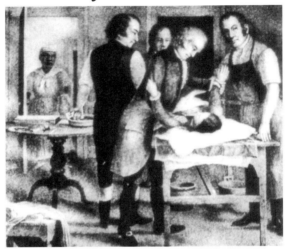

The first ovariotomy, 1809, Danville, Ky.

Discovery and Innovation are perilous — remember Galileo. Perversity is an element of our nature. Changes of mental patterns are resisted ferociously and it is the stuff of strife and conflict. Is it humorous? Yes. The recognition of this facet of ourselves is unsettling, but when it is seen in the long view, it is amusing.

The first great medical innovation in America was the adoption of inoculation to prevent smallpox. The method was discovered in the Middle East, adopted in Turkey, and communicated to Europe in 1714. In 1721 smallpox broke out in Boston and terrified the populace. The Reverend Cotton Mather read of inoculation in a London publication and urged Dr. Zabdiel Boylston of Boston to undertake it.

Dr. Boylston responded. He inoculated his thirteen-year-old son, two other members of his household, and more than a hundred other Bostonians. But Boylston's medical colleagues condemned him and accused him of spreading the disease. Newspapers and pamphlets castigated the practice of inoculation and all those who approved of it. Aroused citizens roamed the town with ropes, threatening to hang Dr. Boylston and a grenade was thrown into the living room of his home. Dr. Boylston had to go into hiding. Everything that could be done was done to obstruct the introduction into America of the first discovered method of preventing smallpox. Dr. Boylston adopted the discovery, demonstrated its usefulness and saved lives. He also demonstrated the perversity of humans that has generated the quip: "No good deed goes unpunished."

Dr. Jesse Bennett seems to have known intuitively that resourcefulness often generates obloquy. In 1794 Dr. Bennett, practicing medicine in the backwoods of Virginia, performed the first successful Cesarean operation in America. When his wife could not deliver their baby he made a desperate effort to save her life and to save the baby. He undertook a Cesarean operation and he saved them both.

A few successful Cesarean operations had been done in Europe. Some babies had been saved, but the mothers did not survive. The operation was so uniformly unsuccessful that it had essentially been abandoned in Europe. Dr. Bennett did not even report his accomplishment. He said that no doctors would believe that this operation could be done successfully in the backwoods of America with the mother surviving, and that he was not going to give anyone the opportunity to call him a liar. One hundred years passed before the first successful Caesarian operation was done in Boston.

Another backwoods American kitchen surgeon made the greatest contribution to the surgical relief of human misery that was made worldwide in the nineteenth century. In 1809

Dr. Ephraim McDowell, a surgeon in Danville, Kentucky, was called to see a woman with a large intra-abdominal tumor, which he recognized as arising from an ovary. The situation was hopeless. Humans did not survive attempts to operate within the abdomen. A slow, agonizing death was the prospect for Dr. McDowell's patient. McDowell told her that if she was prepared to die, he was prepared to attempt to save her. Recognizing integrity, she put herself in his hands. She rode sixty miles on a saddled horse, with the saddle horn chafing against her protuberant abdomen, to McDowell's home in Danville.

At his home in this frontier village, Dr. McDowell strapped his patient's arms and legs to a table in preparation for surgery. There was no anesthesia, she sang hymns and clenched her fists in order to bear the pain as McDowell undertook to remove the tumor.

An angry mob gathered outside the house and demanded that the operation be stopped. The mob swung a rope over a tree limb — it was for McDowell when the patient died. The sheriff restrained some bullies from battering down the door. But McDowell was wise, careful and confident. Experience and contemplation made him think it could be done and he did it. He removed the tumor and after five days his patient was up making her own bed.

McDowell encountered two other patients with the same type of tumor and operated successfully on each of them. Then, in 1817, he wrote an account of his experience for a medical journal. He sent it to the professor of surgery at the University of Pennsylvania who refused to see it published — he did not believe it. When the account was published later, with the assistance of another Philadelphia physician, McDowell was widely denounced — he was called a liar.

The *London Medico-Chirurgical Review*, widely read in Great Britain and the United States, denounced McDowell's claim. The editor asked, how could a surgeon in backwoods America accomplish such a thing? In Scotland the operation was outlawed, and forty years after McDowell cured his first patient, some American professors were still denouncing the operation and seeking to have it forbidden. But McDowell had executed a surgical feat, and his operations had opened the door to abdominal surgery, an epochal medical advance.

Dr. Bennett and Dr. McDowell were fortunate in that the fruition of their ventures at the fringe of medical knowledge did not require the approval or acquiescence of their colleagues or the public. In 1843 when Dr. Oliver Wendell Holmes pushed medicine forward in another of its advances, he was challenging long standing beliefs and practices of his colleagues. That generates resistance, arouses hostility and draws denigration.

Dr. Holmes recognized that childbed fever, a scourge that took the lives of women after childbirth, was an infection caused by inattention to cleanliness on the part of those attending a mother's delivery.

It had been suspected by others, but Holmes, convinced by his own observations, stated that it was so, clearly and authoritatively in a New England medical journal. The scourge could be eliminated, he wrote, if doctors and midwives would change their habits.

Dr. Holmes was denounced. The assault was led by the professor of obstetrics at the Jefferson Medical College in Philadelphia. He was the principal American authority on obstetrics. He insisted that the deaths from childbed fever were due to Providence. His opinion was echoed by the professor of obstetrics at the University of Pennsylvania, who said that doctors could not possibly have a role in the cause of this horrible disease.

But Dr. Holmes was correct. Four years later, Dr. Ignaz Semmelweis, a Hungarian, gathered the statistics to prove it, and history has given him his proper credit. Dr. Holmes shed the criticism that was heaped upon him in the interval and later said he was thankful that life had given him an opportunity to be useful. His was a notable and graceful performance.

When Charles Eliot became president of Harvard University in 1869, he set out to add a new subject to the curriculum of the medical school — bacteriology. It seemed to be a worthy new science, but the opposition was vigorous. Bacteriology was decried as a novelty and was said to have no practical importance. The professor of pediatrics was particularly opposed incorporating it into medicine.

But it was done. And shortly thereafter the organism causing diphtheria — a deadly plague among children — was being identified in the bacteriology laboratory, and an antitoxin to save children's lives was being prepared in the same laboratory. The transition of bacteriology from a field for study to a vital medical auxiliary was remarkably swift — despite the opposition.

In 1886 Dr. Reginald Fitz, in Boston, studied and came to understand how an inflamed appendix caused death, how it could be diagnosed and how it could be treated surgically. It was the greatest triumph of surgery worldwide since McDowell's operation for an ovarian tumor in 1809.

But surgery for appendicitis was much resisted despite the fact that without it, the death rate was 35 percent. In 1890 a Boston medical journal carried an article asserting that Dr. Fitz was in error. Many operations failed because they were resisted until the patient was so stricken that death was inevitable despite surgery.

There followed a period, particularly in small communities, when surgery for appendicitis was tolerated if the patient survived. But if the patient died, a surgeon was likely to be roundly condemned, and the reaction might be so bitter that he would have to move to another place. It finally became clear that surgery was vital and that it was equally vital that the surgery be done early. But acceptance came grudgingly. In 1932, sixteen thousand persons were dying yearly in the United States due to the lack of aggressive surgery. How long does it take for a discovery to become a fact?

When ether anesthesia was discovered and applied to relieve the pain of surgery, it was reasonable to investigate the possibility that ether could be used to alleviate the pains of childbirth. Dr. Walter Channing, professor of obstetrics at Harvard, undertook to do so. In 1848 he wrote that he had collected more than five hundred instances in which ether had been used, and that he was convinced that it was quite helpful in childbirth.

Dr. Channing was pilloried. Mystics asserted that it was morally wrong to alleviate labor pains. Women were supposed to suffer — the Bible said so. Professors of obstetrics agreed. Fortunately, in 1853 Queen Victoria of England accepted anesthesia for the birth of her eighth child. She was so popular in the United States that all opposition to the use of anesthesia in childbirth melted away. It even became fashionable to have anesthesia for childbirth and it was *a la reine*.

In the era of Dr. Holmes and Dr. Channing it proved to be extremely difficult to protect the health of women in childbirth. It did not get easier. Prior to 1850, the female genital area was forbidden territory for doctors and even visual inspection was taboo. But in the 1840s, Dr. Gunning Bedford at the New York University Medical College began to teach gynecology to his students. Cancer of the uterus could often be detected by simple inspection of the vagina and in no other way until it was too late. Dr. Bedford brought a woman before his medical class and demonstrated how to visualize the uterus employing a vaginal speculum. Of course he was denounced, rabidly. The procedure was said to be "an outrage on decency."

Even greater obloquy fell on the head of a professor of obstetrics at the Buffalo Medical College in 1850. He had the temerity to think that medical students might learn best about the birth of a baby by seeing one being born. Doctors were being graduated from medical schools without ever having seen a birth, much less having assisted at one. The professor persuaded an expectant mother to permit a class of students to observe the birth of her baby.

The reaction to this sensible innovation was volcanic. Both the public and the medical profession expressed outrage. The American Medical Association attacked the endeavor. Some medical schools did not provide demonstrations for their students as late as 1890, and even in 1910 many graduating doctors had never seen a normal birth.

Educating the public was even more difficult. In 1937 a group of doctors interested in improving maternal welfare produced an educational film called "The Birth of a Baby." The film was shown at the annual meeting of the American Medical Association. More than four thousand people viewed it at this meeting and there was general hearty approval of the content and purpose of the film. Plans were made to show the film publicly in areas where the local medical societies approved of it and thought it would serve educational purposes.

The first public showing was in Minneapolis. Some two thousand people saw the film in Minneapolis and overwhelmingly approved of it. But in New York the film was banned by the state under laws against obscenity and corruption of morals. In Cincinnati, the city manager tried to block its showing, and Boston censured the film and confiscated an issue of *Life Magazine* that carried picture clips from the film. Obviously, many thought that the people must not see and understand the process of their own reproduction.

In 1902 a medical discovery threatened the dignity of the people of North Carolina and tested their sense of humor. Dr. Charles Stiles of the U.S. Public Health Service demonstrated that almost half of the population of North Carolina harbored hookworms. Americans in the South had long been ravaged by a peculiar disease that caused anemia and sapped their strength. It made them lazy and it was known as the "lazy disease." Newspapers announced that the "germ of laziness" had been found and Dr. Stiles had demonstrated the cause as hookworm.

In 1909 the philanthropic Rockefeller Foundation, aroused by Dr. Stiles' discovery, created a commission to study hookworm disease and combat it. The project should have been hailed by rejoicing, but it was not. Instead the governor of North Carolina said it was an effort by "a bunch of Yankees... trying to intimidate us Southerners into thinking we have hookworms... I'm telling you there is no such thing." A Tampa, Florida, paper suggested that Dr. Stiles should be lynched.

The worm is acquired when one goes barefoot on contaminated soil. The first stage of the disease, slow-healing sores on the feet, was called "dew p'izen," in the South. When people were told that they must wear shoes to prevent hookworm disease, they said that Rockefeller was going into the shoe business and this was a scheme to get them to wear shoes all year long.

But in one campaign in North Carolina, of 320,000 people examined, 160,000 were found to harbor the worms. The facts destroyed the denials.

Drives were launched to eliminate hookworm in the South and they succeeded — drugs can clear the intestinal tract of the worms and shoes prevent re-infection and new cases. The campaign was a great success. By 1927 hookworm disease was all but wiped out. Public pride denied the Rockefeller Foundation its proper credit. In 1967 an elderly Tar Heel was reminded of these events and he responded, "I doubt if there ever was such a thing as hookworm."

In 1905 Dr. William Osler demonstrated how even proposing (or being thought to propose) an innovation can provoke a furious reaction. Dr. Osler was the professor of medicine at the Johns Hopkins University and the most respected and revered figure in American medicine. When he retired from his post, a grand farewell dinner was given in Baltimore, and Dr. Osler addressed his friends for the last time. He called his address "The Fixed Period." He said that most men have done their best work, made their greatest contributions to society by the time they are forty, and that science, commerce, and government would benefit if men were retired at sixty.

Unfortunately, Osler took the title for his address from a novel by Anthony Trollope in which a group of men anticipating their decline agreed to be chloroformed at the age of sixty. Osler did not endorse any such action, but the press dubbed his talk the Chloroform Address, and reported that he did. The word "Oslerize" was coined to describe it. A national storm broke over Osler's head and threatening letters poured in "by the wagon load" from all over the country. Dr. Osler, an accomplished, humble and generous man, retired in a torrent of abuse — all of it unjust and misdirected.

There is an axiom in physics that seems equally applicable to human endeavors: For every action there is an equal and opposite reaction. Dr. George King, who practiced on Long Island through the early 1900s, recalled how some of his patients reacted when he adopted new techniques for their benefit. When rubber gloves were introduced, Dr. King wore them during deliveries to protect his patients from infection. But some women resented his wearing them: "Thinks he's too darned good to handle me with his bare hands," one said. "Guess he's afraid he'll catch something."

The first American attempts to ameliorate heart disease by surgery were made in the early 1900s. They were directed at a heart valve that is commonly deformed in childhood by inflammation due to rheumatic fever. The heart damage leads to death years later in the prime of life. The first attempts failed and surgery was abandoned.

In Philadelphia, in 1948, Dr. Charles Bailey thought that he had conceived a better surgical technique for reaching the involved heart valve and correcting its deformity. He operated on three patients, but they all died. Because of these failures, three of the five hospitals in Philadelphia refused to let Dr. Bailey do any more heart valve operations.

Dr. Bailey was undeterred. He scheduled a fourth and a

fifth operation on the same day, one in the morning and one in the afternoon. He would do one operation at each of the two hospitals that had not yet refused him the use of their operating rooms. He knew that if these operations failed, the two remaining hospitals would also surely close their doors to him. He planned to have a taxi waiting, and if the fourth operation failed he would hurry to the next hospital before the news got out and any action could be taken against him to prevent a fifth attempt.

Dr. Bailey's determination bordered on the irrational. Why would he persist? What if he was mistaken? Was this a ruthless quest for recognition or a tenacious dedication to a perceived insight? Dr. Bailey also wondered: "You know that almost all the world is against it. You know you have a great personal stake and might even lose your medical license or at least hospital privileges if you persist. In fact, the thought crosses your mind that maybe you really are crazy. And yet you feel that it has to be done."

The fourth operation failed and the patient died in surgery. Bailey raced to the hospital of last resort and did the fifth operation. The fifth operation succeeded. The road to successful heart surgery was opened and it has been extended ever since.

Men with this sort of intensity generate some very strong feelings among their fellow doctors and may generate animosity that smolders for a lifetime. Chicago surgeon John B. Murphy induced record-setting disapproval.

Dr. Murphy was one of the eminent surgeons of his era. He was successively the professor of surgery at Northwestern University and at the Rush Medical College in Chicago between 1901 and 1916. Dr. William Mayo called him "the surgical genius of our generation." He was a peerless teacher, a prodigious worker, and a man who received boundless acclaim from his patients for his courtesy and kindness. But Dr. Murphy's colleagues disliked him. They thought him arrogant and excessively self-promotional. When Dr. Murphy was proposed for membership in an elite Chicago medical-social society, he was rejected.

Sixteen years after Dr. Murphy's death, a member of the same Chicago society thought that Murphy deserved better. Time had shown that the society had rejected a good man. The mistake should be acknowledged and Dr. Murphy should be admitted posthumously to erase the error. He proposed Dr. Murphy for membership and when the vote was taken — seventeen years after his death — Murphy was rejected again.

Wiser men can recognize professional merit in their colleagues and separate it from their personal tastes and some can do it with wit and good humor. One of the country's great surgeons was characterized in this vein by a colleague: "I didn't like him a damn bit, but I admired him tremendously." And there is the witty judgment of the physician who was told that a well-known professor was moving from Harvard to Yale and asked his opinion of the move. He replied that he approved of it. He said that he thought it would raise the academic level of both institutions.

When Dr. Alton Ochsner proposed the creation of a medical clinic in New Orleans after the model of the Mayo Clinic, he aroused no enthusiasm and much opposition from his medical colleagues. But in 1939 five doctors joined him and the group persuaded a bank to finance the establishment of the Ochsner Clinic in a remodeled building. Clinics compete with private practitioners for patients and this gives rise to tensions. On Good Friday 1941 each of the founders of the Ochsner Clinic had delivered to the door of his home a small leather pouch with thirty dimes ("pieces of silver") in it and an anonymous note that read:

"To the Judases of the New Orleans Medical Society."

In Boston Dr. Ernest Codman suffered similar mindless hostility in the same period. It is humorous only in retrospect. Dr .Codman, an astute and restless innovator, was interested in diseases of the shoulder. His opinions and new surgical procedures met the usual dissent and opposition. In the preface of one of his books he described the effect that an innovative mindset can have on its possessor.

"Through much of my life I have suffered somewhat from a sense of isolation because I have always been thinking, or saying, one thing or another with which other doctors did not agree. This, in my early years, made me suspect myself of being peculiar, so that from time to time I would conform again to general opinions which I knew to be irrational.... I have become more and more content to wait for the acceptance of my views. My regrets are for wasting so much time on the opinions of a previous generation and not realizing that it was the approval of my pupils, rather than of my masters, that was desirable.... Now my pleasure comes from having younger men agree to ideas that which my contemporaries rejected."

Aside from his interest in surgery of the shoulder, Dr. Codman had questions about the end results of all surgery. How did operations turn out? Which ones were effective and which ones were not?

No one took the trouble to find out. He called it the "End Result Idea." He queried all of his patients after one year to determine if the result of their surgery was good or inadequate. He urged other Boston surgeons to do the same, but there was no response.

To make his point, Dr. Codman resigned from the staff of the Massachusetts General Hospital.

After his resignation had been accepted, he wrote to the hospital and in an ironical jest asked to be appointed surgeon-in-chief on the grounds that his result were better than those of any other surgeon in Boston.

There could be no dispute because there could be no comparison. No other surgeon had followed his patients to ascertain the results. His request was ignored and he was regarded as a nuisance.

Dr. Codman took his idea to a meeting of the medical

society where he presented it formally and forcefully. He suggested that all surgical cases be reviewed after one year to determine the effectiveness of the surgery. Then he suggested that money might be the reason that the idea was so strongly resisted. Perhaps some surgeons did not want to know because some operations might have to be abandoned and this would reduce surgical income.

The result was disastrous. Dr. Codman lost friends, was excluded socially by most doctors, was asked to resign as chairman of the medical society, was dropped from the Harvard medical staff and his income fell precipitately.

The American College of Surgeons subsequently took up the idea of following surgical patients to determine and compare long-term results, and today every medical center does it routinely to assess the effectiveness of what has been done and compare it with new innovative procedures.

Medical research is now a costly enterprise requiring expensive apparatus, laboratories, and teams of scientists. Two new players are on the stage: the two who hold the purse-strings, the philanthropic foundations and the government. They add new facets of perversity to the comedies of discovery and innovation.

In 1931 Dr. Alvin Coburn suspected that "strep throat" infections in children increased the likelihood of subsequent rheumatic fever which in turn often causes heart damage. He published his thesis and some preliminary supporting data. Shortly thereafter, Dr. Coburn was "invited" to call on an established and distinguished medical investigator who was interested in rheumatic fever, and who was supported by a wealthy foundation. Dr. Coburn was told that his research was deceptively conceived and presented, and that if he persisted in his course he would be exposed as a charlatan. Any such criticism from such a source would terminate Coburn's career in academia, and this was exactly what his detractor meant to convey. Dr. Coburn wrote, "It was one of the most devastating days of my life."

That was enough, but a second censor undertook to de-nounce Dr. Coburn to the Surgeon General's office on one occasion and to the National Institutes of Health on another when Coburn applied for funds for research. The latter attack was oral and so ferocious that a friend who heard it and told Coburn about it asked facetiously, "Have you ever assaulted his wife?"

Dr. Coburn's intuition proved to be correct. The inci-dence of heart damage due to rheumatic fever in children has been reduced by aggressive treatment of "strep throat" infections.

In 1620 Francis Bacon, the eminent philosopher of sci-ence, wrote, "It would be an unsound fancy and self contra-dictory to expect that things which have never been done can be done except by means which have never yet been tried." Will we ever attend to this dictum?

The first effective treatment for breast cancer was surgical. It was an extensive operation involving removal of the breast along with adjacent lymph nodes and chest muscles. The operation was devised in 1894 and was the recommended treatment for breast cancer for the following fifty years.

In the 1940s some surgeons reported experiences suggest-ing that simple breast removal followed by irradiation therapy was just as effective as the more extensive surgery. Dr. George Crile Jr. of the Cleveland Clinic pursued this idea and in 1935 he published a popular book advocating the less aggressive sur-gery. Professional opposition was vehement and concordant. *Life Magazine* asked Dr. Crile to write a synopsis of the book, and when it was ready *Life* sent a pre-publication copy to the American Cancer Society for review. The result was that the American Cancer Society tried to block the publication of the piece. When this failed, they settled for a banner of dis-sent across the title page: "A Statement Disagreeing With Dr. Crile," which was signed by the president of the American Medical Association, the director of the National Cancer Institute and the director of the American Cancer Society.

Of Dr. Crile, they said, "His thesis is contrary to the teaching of the country's 81 medical schools and to the experience of physicians and surgeons."

They did not say it should be studied further and they did not say that Dr. Crile was not alone in this opinion. They simply said it was contrary to established opinion and therefore in error. They re-enacted the condemnation of Galileo. It was as though Francis Bacon had not lived.

Dr. Crile and a few other surgeons came to believe that the breast did not have to be removed — only the tumor. In Boston Dr. Oliver Cope was also persuaded that the breast did not have to be removed and published his opinion in 1970. He repeated it in a book published in 1978. The *Boston Globe* reported that the reaction to Dr. Cope's views — almost a quarter of a century after the Crile contretemps — "varied from frosty to furious." Dr. Cope and a colleague were called before the Massachusetts Medical Society to explain why they were not doing the old operation. Resistance was staunch over all these years.

But in 1979 a conference of cancer specialists at the National Institutes of Health supported the views that Drs. Crile and Cope had espoused courageously despite much disparagement over many years. These tales exemplify a whimsical paradox that is an element of our nature: The greatest hindrance to learning something new is what we already "know." Mark Twain put it more amusingly: "It isn't what you don't know that will hurt you, it's what you do know that isn't so."

The scientific method o'er-leaps such barriers to knowledge and discovery. But one must learn to discover not by trying to prove things, but by disproving alternatives. This is laborious. Discovery is difficult. It is estimated that there are unwarranted conclusions — errors — in two-thirds of the studies published in our best medical journals. Progress is slow. Serendipity and intuition have no role. The only abiding directive is THINK and try an experiment.

16.
The Realm of the Self

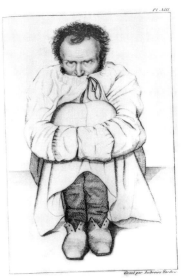

The Realm of the Self is the last great frontier of medicine. Disorders of the brain are little understood and the genesis of behavior eludes scientific study. Philosophers contend that a brain can never understand itself. Nonetheless, it is our destiny to pursue the mystery of the mind, and we may ultimately gain some insight into ourselves. If we do, we will surely confirm that a sense of humor is one of our elementary attributes.

Astonishingly, humor commonly flashes forth even from the minds of persons who are severely demented. I recall a young lady confined to a mental institution who greeted me in a smiling, friendly manner each time we met, and always with the same salutation: "Hello doctor," she said. "How's your schizophrenia, megalomania, dementia, paranoia today?" And without waiting for an answer, she laughed and added: "When you can joke about your insanity, that's a sign you are getting well." She had been in the hospital for twelve years and she was not improving.

A thirty-five-year-old who came under my care in the same institution had been committed to the hospital permanently to prevent self-mutilation. Her arms, legs, and neck were covered with the scars from great lacerations, self-inflicted over a number of years. Each time I met her and asked her how she was getting along, she replied: "Fine Doc, I'm not cutting up."

And a man with extensive and hopeless brain damage due to syphilis used to put his hand on my shoulder when we met. He was about 5'2" and had done some boxing at one time. "Doc," he said, "with my brains and your body we could win the heavyweight championship."

In the American Colonies the mentally afflicted were cared for by their families, or in the almshouses along with the poor, or occasionally, if they were violent, they were restrained in some especially devised strong-room. Treatment, when any was offered, was based on folklore or derived from superstition. The Reverend Cotton Mather advised prayer and fasting for madness. At that time disease was regarded as due to sin, and madness due to diabolical possession. Mather believed in such treatments as cutting a roasted bird in two and placing it, reeking hot, on the head of a demented person. German colonists in Pennsylvania thought that madness was due to the "haernfresser," a fanciful insect that entered the brain through the ear.

The first hospital in America was established in Philadelphia in 1751. One of the two patients admitted on the opening day was a "lunatic."

Doctors knew nothing about the causes of insanity or the varieties of madness. Lunatic was a simple, all-inclusive designation. Subsequently the Pennsylvania Hospital took in an "outrageous person." Another early patient was described as an "irregular person." There was one who was found naked in the streets — thus not requiring any singular description — and some who had become "a terror to their neighbors." These were the definitions of madness and the extent of knowledge.

Treatment was primarily custodial, but it included bleeding and purging as was done for most other afflictions in that era. Blistering, in the case of the insane, was done on the scalp. Dr. Benjamin Rush, who cared for the insane in this first hospital in Philadelphia, is regarded as the "father of American psychiatry."

From the beginning, the mentally disturbed provided moments of diversion. "Polly" was among the troubled persons taken into the Pennsylvania Hospital. One day in the course of her stay, a large crowd assembled at a "bull baiting" a short way from the hospital. At a bull baiting, a wild bull was taunted by dogs and men, inside a small fenced arena, in a manner similar to a Spanish bullfight. A bull that had just destroyed several dogs and tossed a man violently was looking for a new challenger when Polly — straying from the hospital — came over the high fence and into the ring.

She was without shoes, "bosom all open, her neck bare and her beautiful ringlets wildly dangling over her shoulders — her other clothing was her shift only and a white petticoat." She went straight to the bull and stroked its head murmuring, "Are they hurting you?"

The spectators were breathless and transfixed. No one dared enter the ring to rescue Polly. But the bull dropped his head and became gentle. Suddenly Polly darted away, scaled the fence again and scampered back to the hospital.

Another patient at the Pennsylvania Hospital escaped from his ward and made his way to the roof where he barricaded himself in a cupola and successfully defied all attempts to dislodge him. The effort was finally abandoned, and his clothing and bedding were brought up and given to him. He lived in his rooftop cupola for nine years — until his death — surviving nine Philadelphia winters without heat. He was sort of an original homeless person, a refugee from the asylum.

In 1773 Virginia became the first state to establish a "lunatic asylum," and it was the only state to support such an institution before 1810. But by 1860 twenty-eight of the thirty-three states had public asylums. This development was not associated with any increased understanding of insanity. Its object was primarily to maintain peace and order by taking the wandering insane — those for whom no one took responsibility — off the streets and to provide custodial care for those who could not be cared for at home. But it represented the acceptance of a new idea. Madness was removed from the realms of folklore, religion, and superstition and recognized to be a medical problem.

The doctors who superintended the new asylums learned a great lesson that was subsequently forgotten: that many of the people in these institutions led useful and contented lives in a hospital though they were incapable of getting along outside of it. Dr. William A. White, superintendent of Saint Elizabeth's Hospital in Washington, D.C., from 1903 to 1937, described it as a place "where one has a right to be queer. One may say queer things and do queer things without being looked at askance and without being made fun of... the tension these people suffer outside is removed when they get adjusted to their new life in the hospital."

Dr. White enjoyed citing examples. He told of an inmate who was a skilled tinsmith and who worked efficiently with the hospital plumbers and steamfitters. He never spoke. He pretended to read for long periods, but he could not read and often held his book upside down. Each day he walked off the grounds for a distance of about three miles, a mallet in hand, stood before a Soldier's Monument, rapped his mallet on the railing surrounding the monument and "reported." On one occasion when a fellow worker was injured he ran to an adjacent building and spoke precisely about the need for help — the only time he was known to speak. He troubled no one.

An asylum might even provide a sense of security to a troubled person. Dr. White described a typical asylum ward with rooms opening on a central corridor, each room with a single barred window. In one room at the end of the corridor an attendant was on duty twenty-four hours a day and the window was not barred. A hospital reorganization eliminated the permanent attendant in favor of a roving supervisor and the vacated room was offered to a well-behaved patient. It was a desirable room, and he seemed pleased to get it. But on the first night that he occupied his new room he picked up his blanket and pillow in the middle of the night and moved back to his previous quarters. When he was asked why, he replied, "You don't expect me to sleep in a room where there are no bars on the windows."

Of his patients, Dr. White wrote: "I learned that many of these people, as crazy as they were to use the ordinary lay term, were nevertheless fine characters, in many instances far more reliable than the average person one meets outside." And after a lifetime of experience, Dr. White added: "I have always felt that some of the best friends I have ever had were among the patients in the institutions for mental disease.... I make this comment... because I know how incomprehensible such a statement is to the average person."

It is a truism often forgotten that the mentally disturbed are much more like the rest of us than different from us. Dr. White told of a well-known literary figure who advertised in the supplements of Sunday newspapers requesting information on the origin, meaning and usage of obscure words. He was editing a great new dictionary. One person answered the ads repeatedly and always supplied information that was helpful. This correspondent came to be so highly regarded by the editor that he wrote and invited his correspondent to lunch. He wanted to meet him. The correspondent replied that he would be unable to come, but he would be pleased to have the editor visit him instead.

The editor, James Murray, who was editing the Oxford English Dictionary, did make a visit. He even took his wife along anticipating a very interesting afternoon. They probably were a little unnerved when they found themselves in front of a mental asylum, but they proceeded and had a pleasant visit with a fellow word maven who had been in the asylum for years and never recovered.

This same theme received an update in 1953. The Army journal *Military Review* published an article on the peril of handheld nuclear weapons. They were theoretically feasible and terrorists would be empowered by them. The journal was published at the army's Command and General Staff College in Fort Leavenworth, Kansas, and was circulated to some nineteen thousand senior officers and foreign subscribers. The editors reviewed the facts of the piece carefully, but were less attentive to the status of the author. After publication, it was discovered that the author was confined to a Tennessee asylum and had been there for nine years.

The boundary where sanity shades into insanity is vague. The line is arbitrary and judgments can be difficult to make. The White House in Washington becomes a focus of many disturbed minds. They journey to the capital from all across the country to tell the president about such things as aliens in space who are directing harmful rays to their bodies and about fantastic plots directed against themselves and against the nation. The Secret Service is alert to the problem and skillful at detecting and dealing with it. When such visitors are stopped at the White House gate and judged to be disturbed they are whisked off to the government asylum for disposition.

One day a gentle little lady from rural North Carolina was brought to the asylum by the Secret Service. She had appeared at the White House gate with a cake for the president. She had baked it herself and traveled from North Carolina to present it. She was a simple, good-hearted person unaware that there would be any problem associated with bringing a gift to her president. The police thought her errand was irrational. There was nothing the matter with her and she was released from the hospital immediately,

As the insane were gathered into public asylums in the first half of the nineteenth century, it became apparent that a very large group of people who were not insane complained of disturbances that seemed to be related to the brain. They complained of depression, insomnia, weakness, tremulousness, inexplicable fears, obsessive thoughts, fluttering hearts, and ungovernable stomachs. They complained of "nervousness."

Knowledge regarding nervousness was also nil. It seemed to be a new human disorder. In 1869 an American neurologist Dr. George Beard gathered all of these symptoms — everything short of blatant insanity — into one new concept, a new disease. He called it neurasthenia. He said it was an American disease caused by the climate and the pace of life in America. He wrote a book called *American Nervousuesa*. He feared that American nervousness was increasing rapidly, and indeed it did seem to increase. Dr. Beard said that he suffered from neurasthenia himself and that one-third of his patients were doctors. The treatment was bed rest, sedation, soothing baths and electrical stimulation.

But neurasthenia was only a conglomeration of symptoms tagged with a euphonious name. It was a composite of unknowns, not an entity, but it was a spectrum of obscure disturbances. A perceptive contemporary neurologist called it: "A condition known through a feat of the imagination." It was the disease of living.

But Dr. Weir Mitchell, a Philadelphia neurologist, gave neurasthenia an unfortunate legitimacy and devised a Rest Cure for it that became a fad. The cure consisted of isolation and complete bed rest. Only the doctor and a nurse saw the patient. Even mail was disallowed. A fattening, dairy product diet was given along with massage and electrotherapy. After six to eight weeks of the rest cure, patients were pronounced cured, allowed up, and some were indeed much improved — temporarily. Thousands were treated.

Most neurasthenics were women. Occasionally one would not get up when the cure was said to be over. Dr. Mitchell ordered one woman to get up and she refused; she said she was not well yet. But the treatment was over, she must get up. Dr. Mitchell told her that if she remained in bed he would get into bed with her, but she still refused. The doctor took off his coat and vest as if to carry out his threat, but the woman was adamant. Dr. Mitchell proceeded to unbutton his pants and the woman scampered out of bed.

Dr. Mitchell had prevailed by layering humbug on humbug in a performance fit only for a circus tent.

This was the milieu when psychoanalysis appeared on the scene. Freudianism came to America at the turn of the century. The insane were in the asylums and labeled psychotic. The less disturbed — the victims of neurasthenia — were labeled neurotic, and were to be the beneficiaries of psychoanalysis. Dr. Freud claimed to have discovered the cause of neurotic behavior in the memories of his patients. His disciples applied these discoveries to explain human development, disease states, history, art, literature and corporate practices. They even explained why critics of psychoanalysis were critical — thereby annihilating criticism. Neurasthenia disappeared. Neurosis replaced it and psychoanalysis replaced bed rest and warm baths.

What was psychoanalysis? A sect with such grandiose pretensions acquired and deserved some witty definitions. A Jewish doctor said it was "a specialty for Jewish doctors who were afraid of the sight of blood." It was said to be "a way to correct our faults by confessing our parents' shortcomings." Some said it was "an accredited method by which a man may have an indecent conversation with a decent woman." Critics said, "It isn't medicine it's literature," or "It isn't science, it's ideology."

The psychoanalysts required that a doctor be analyzed before being recognized as a qualified analyst. This canon led to such comedies as one in which an analyst was seeing twenty-six patients two to five times weekly — treating them — while seeing his own analyst five times a week. Amused observers pictured themselves being treated by an analyst who was seeing an analyst, who was seeing an analyst, who was seeing an analyst, who was...

Jesters spoofed psychoanalysis as the only medical specialty in which doctors have to undergo five years of treatment (analysis) before they could practice. This requirement was compared to having to have cancer before one could be a cancer specialist, or having to die before one could be a proper pathologist.

Psychoanalysis was an expensive, time-consuming endeavor directed at people who were minimally ill. Often they were not ill at all and better described as the "worried well." It completely ignored the asylum population. The treatment was not suited to them. This reversed the usual order of things in which the most complex and expensive treatment is directed at the most complex and troublesome disorders. It is astonishing to realize what was proclaimed as a breakthrough in the comprehension of mental mechanisms had no application to the people whose mental mechanisms were the most disordered.

The Freudians asserted that neurotic disorders (neurasthenia) stemmed from psychic traumas of infancy: distressing experiences, including the distress of being born. This was wildly speculative. It was an invitation to satirists, and satirists had great fun with it.

One wit suggested that the concept of birth as psychic trauma created an obvious need for preventive psychotherapy. He proposed that every fetus receive psychoanalytic counseling during the last few weeks before delivery. The counseling would deal first with the anxiety the fetus would have about the forthcoming event. The analyst would explain the nature of the delivery and allay concerns about the stress involved and the risks incurred. The counseling would be given with the mother positioned so that the fetus was reclining — the counterpart to adult therapy in which the patient reclined on a couch. During the counseling period the primal scene (psychoanalytic jargon for sexual congress) should not be acted or the fetus would witness it and suffer psychic trauma.

Humorists discerned that the birth process sometimes confirmed another psychoanalytic concept. Occasionally, when twins are born, one twin emerges with the umbilical cord wrapped tightly around its neck. With the benefit of psychoanalytic insight, this circumstance, which had long been regarded as incidental, could now be correctly interpreted as intense sibling rivalry — begun in the womb — and measures to counter it were instituted immediately.

Physicians were indoctrinated with such notions as the Oedipus complex, castration anxiety, penis envy, and the anal and oral phases of child development. Enthusiasm for these inventions swept up most, though not all, psychiatrists. When students discussed the psychoanalytic concepts of human development at the Johns Hopkins University in the 1940s, Dr. Leo Kanner, professor of child psychiatry suggested that they add a "pharyngeal phase" to the sequence of development. He said it was a phase in which one would swallow anything.

Another jester pointed out that Dr. Freud had overlooked a structure that plays a major role in a baby's first experiences. The mouth and the anus are important, but what about the nose? When a child is born, the first thing it experiences is the fussing of doctors and nurses at its nose — clearing it of mucous. This nasal trauma must make a very powerful impression on a child. It could well be responsible for the development of a nose-centered personality — a concept that psychoanalysts had not explored.

The features of a nose-centered personality come readily to mind. The size of the nose would doubtless be important.

Nose-centered children with large noses would very likely become aggressive, develop a tendency to stick their noses into other people's business, and to look down their noses at their fellows. Such arrogance might lead to guilt feelings, which, in turn, would lead them to have their noses made smaller by plastic surgeons.

Psychoanalysts were not amused. Worse, they rejected such humor — all humor. A prominent psychoanalyst wrote that humor was destructive in psychotherapy and it should never enter into psychoanalytic relationships. His colleagues made it official. The publisher of a humorous periodical spoofing psychologists and psychiatrists exhibited his magazine at the annual meetings of the American Psychiatric Association and the American Psychological Association. He was seeking recognition and new subscribers as many publishers do. He wanted to display and promote his publication at the annual meeting of the American Psychoanalytic Association as well, but the psychoanalysts rejected his request. A representative declared that humor had no place in psychoanalysis.

It is curious that psychoanalysis chose to be humorless. Freud defined psychotherapy as "talking people into and out of things." The humorist Leo Rosten defined humor as "the affectionate communication of insight." The definitions beg to be blended. Might psychotherapy be fruitfully defined as talking people into and out of things through the affectionate communication of insight?

In the course of therapy, psychiatrists listen and listen, and much of what they listen to is boring. One psychiatrist complained that some of his patients didn't even have interesting fantasies.

A principal psychiatric journal featured an article on the problem of boring patients. The piece dealt specifically with problems such as how to avoid thinking about lunch rather than listening to the patient. Satirists took the clue and carried the idea to its limits. One imagined two psychiatrist who rode down in an elevator at the end of a day. One was fresh and eager, squash racket in hand, ready to polish off his day in a contest at the gym. The other was visibly tired and drooping — finished. "How can you be so fresh," he asked, "after listening to these tales of anguish all day?" His fellow psychiatrist responded: "Who listens?"

And indeed a psychiatrist could be effective without listening and lunch might even play a role. A young man in his thirties told of being burdened by a great sense of hopelessness. He consulted a psychiatrist and proceeded to see him weekly. After several sessions, there came a day when as the young man was talking, the psychiatrist, who had just come from lunch, burped. The young man continued to talk, but he was haunted by that burp.

Driving home, he recollected the scene and burst into laughter at the thought of it. He laughed so much that tears came to his eyes and he had to pull his car over to the curb. He said, "I was feeling utterly dejected, alone and devoid of hope — and he burped!" The burp put an entirely new perspective on things. The young man cancelled his future appointments, thanked the psychiatrist for his help and went on his way entirely free of his woe.

Psychoanalysis swept over America. By the 1940s it dominated American psychiatry. When psychoanalysis was embraced, psychiatry divorced itself from biology. The "psyche" was a metaphor and it had no anatomy, physiology or chemistry. A psychiatrist at the Massachusetts General Hospital described the result. In 1945 the psychiatrists ceased to carry stethoscopes. Then they ceased to wear identifying medical white coats. By 1955 they had ceased to attend the hospital's medical conferences. Psychiatrists generally stopped doing physical examinations on their patients. Psychiatry was de-medicalized. The mind was divorced from the brain as thoroughly as when Aristotle located it in the heart.

The divorce from biology opened two grand avenues of folly. First, the problems of life became diseases to be treated and behavior was labeled illness. The ills of the spirit and the distresses of the human situation became psychiatric disorders. Addictions, delinquency, promiscuity, and antisocial attitudes and actions were added to the list. Everyone could be seen as a little mad.

Simultaneously, the divorce from medicine encouraged the proliferation of fanciful, non-biological therapies. There came to be more than three hundred and fifty forms of psychotherapy. There was dance therapy, art therapy, psychodrama, music therapy, assertive training and stress reduction, to name just a few. A skeptical medical educator observed that some of the therapies required a therapist who was as irrational as the patients.

The Freudians proclaimed that unhappy experiences were repressed into an unconscious and that such repression caused mental and physical distress. But the unconscious is an abstraction and a critical, discerning psychiatrist called it an "imaginary cesspool." Nonetheless, it quickly came to be regarded as a reality.

The psychoanalysts probed the minds of their patients for troublesome thoughts buried in the unconscious. Reluctance to discuss a topic was said to mean that it was painful and was a signal for the analyst to pursue it with redoubled intensity. This interpretation might produce some mortifying results.

A woman who heard voices, when questioned by her psychiatrist, said that she heard two voices, At times she heard a pleasant voice and at times she was addressed by scornful, mocking voice. "Are you hearing them now?" the psychiatrist asked. "Yes," she replied, she was hearing the mocking voice. "And what does it say?" the psychiatrist asked. "I'd rather not tell you," she responded and the questioner countered with, "Go ahead. I'm a doctor. You can tell me anything." "Well," she offered, "It's saying don't pay any attention to that big mutton-head. He doesn't know anything and he can't help you."

The transformation of the problems of life into diseases to be treated raised some puzzling questions. Psychiatrists saw many of their own personal problems in their patients and some wondered: Where does the doctor end and the patient begin? Young doctors learning to be psychiatrists were given the most disturbed patients so that they would have less difficulty making the distinction. Patients also wondered. A psychiatrist wrote, "The patient enters my office dubious of his own sanity and departs dubious of mine." Psychiatrists became wary of getting too close to their colleagues for the same reason. Revealing too much about one's self, they said could turn one into a patient. A tale circulated about a pigeon flying into the meeting hall at a convention of psychiatrists. No one paid any attention to the pigeon. No psychiatrist was willing to be the first to say that he saw a pigeon fly in through the window.

Psychoanalysis was greatly oversold. The expectation that persons could be made over by psychoanalysis proved to be untenable and it could not be done. When this became clear, the goal of treatment became crisis management: Deal with the current problem and stop there. Psychoanalysis degraded to counseling. A Harvard neurologist offered a properly scaled down definition: "It is 90 percent common sense and 10 percent German nonsense." It was counseling, guidance provided with equal effectiveness by a friend, a clergyman, a teacher or a family doctor.

Perceptive patients shed the mystique even when they benefited from the process. A good-natured girl who had allowed a preoccupation with a mild curvature of her upper spine to impair her self-image wrote an amusing thank you note to her psychoanalyst after she improved:

> *For analysis I'll always vouch*
> *It reduced my 'hunch' to a slouch*
> *Was this due to lost fears?*
> *Or simply to the years*
> *I lay flat on my back on the couch?*

Critics coined cautionary aphorisms that dissipated the analytic aura: "Never go to a psychiatrist who analyzes a joke instead of laughing at it;" and "Beware of the psychiatrist who goes to the Follies Bergere and watches the audience."

By 1960 psychoanalysis was in severe decline and there was a professional consensus that it was ill conceived. A Nobel Prize winning biologist said of it: "Its ruins... will remain forever one of the saddest and strangest of all landmarks in the history of twentieth century thought." Some summaries were bitter. One said that Sigmund Freud would be remembered in the category that included Hans Christian Anderson and the Grimm brothers.

Then what could one do with the burden of life? Psychiatrist William Welch summed it up.

1. *There was religiosity: Be solaced by a life of good works.*
2. *Philosophy: Rely on faith in the mind.*
3. *Asceticism: Seek the way.*
4. *Worry: Accept recurrent dissatisfaction.*
5. *Achieve: Diversion by accomplishment.*

The goal is called salvation, knowledge, consciousness, enlightenment, satori, nirvana etc. Make a choice. It is the human situation.

Psychiatrists scrambled to find a new basis for the study of mental disorders. One group created Social Psychiatry. They said that human neurotic dysfunctions were due to our social system and would never be alleviated until poverty, social inequality and poor education were eliminated. This was psychiatry's proper objective. Some even added world peace to the agenda. The idea was extraordinary. Having failed with individuals, psychiatrists were to treat communities. They were not fitted for the task and this venture failed.

Another reformist group asserted that human behavior, neuroses, addiction, crime and social dysfunction should be a field of study entirely divorced from medical psychiatry

— the care of the insane. Separate new schools should be established to study behavior, they said.

A third group contended that the entire concept of mental disease was erroneous — there is no such thing. The psyche is a metaphor and a metaphor cannot be sick. Psychiatric labels, they said, were simply designations for socially unacceptable behavior and socially unacceptable behavior was cultural. It was fluid and it changed with time and society, This movement was called anti-psychiatry,

In summary, psychiatry had fragmented into chaos. A dean of the specialty wrote that, "psychiatry rides madly in all directions." It was going nowhere. At least five thousand papers were published on schizophrenia between 1920 and 1966 and nothing of therapeutic significance had come of it.

What were young people — students and residents — who contemplated becoming psychiatrists to think of all this? They were confused and distressed. If psychotherapy was simply counseling, some cynics saw its elaboration as "stabilizing patients by love" or, from a patient's view, "the purchase of friendship." A dismayed psychiatric resident said: "We're all gigolos."

Trainees were offered some guidance in 1974 in a publication titled *A Survival Guide for Psychiatric Residents.* The guide suggested that since psychiatry was in chaos, one solution for a trainee was to reverse course and become a pediatrician or a radiologist. Or one could make a lateral move into research or administration. Or a fledgling could conclude that since nobody seemed to know anything reliable about psychiatry he could "wing it," that is, resort to what was called "Guts Therapy:" Do anything that seemed to be appropriate for the moment, ranging from stroking to screaming — some doctors actually prescribed screaming sessions. And lastly there was the "Afghanistan-Nepal-Marrakech Sidestep," in which one not only removed himself from psychiatry, but also from the Western World, concluding that psychiatry will never answer the questions that confront it and seeking enlightenment in Eastern mystical experience.

Beginning in 1950 drug therapy for psychiatric disorders produced some striking results. This approach expanded rapidly and today it dominates psychiatry. It has brought psychiatry back into medicine. Armed with drugs, the psychiatrists have donned white coats again, acquired stethoscopes, and rejoined the medical doctors at hospital conferences.

The role of drugs in the treatment of mental disturbances is yet to be defined. Mental disabilities associated with diseases are likely to yield to some degree to this approach. It is likely that the problems of living — depression, insecurity, hostility and self-destructiveness — will not. It has been remarked that the chemistry that produces socially harmonious thoughts is the same chemistry that produces hostile and destructive ideas.

Neurasthenia is still with us. Today it is most commonly called "nerves." Sophisticated parlance describes it as "stress," or perhaps "burnout," or the "chronic fatigue syndrome." These are manifestations of the soul/mind complex, a realm that despite much investigation remains closed to our understanding.

Index

97, 105, 118, 119, 120,
150, 155, 156, 169,
175, 178, 181, 183,
193, 216, 223, 226,
228, 232, 233, 236
Boston City Hospital 77, 80,
85, 150, 169
Boston Globe 236
Boston Medical and Surgical
Journal 99
Boylston, Zabdiel 223
Brooklyn Bridge 198
Buffalo Medical College 227
Bulkeley, Gershom 126
Burlington, Vermont 143
Burnum, John 195
Burr, Joseph S. 162

C

Cabot, Richard 68
California, state of 51, 100,
102, 160
Calvinism 11
Canada 89
Cape May 129
Cardiff, Wales 216
Castleton, Vermont 24
Cattell, Richard 82
Channing, Walter 227
Charleston, South Carolina
106
Chicago, Illinois 16, 39, 44,
47, 59, 76, 96, 105,
110, 118, 124, 127,
129, 136, 179, 190,
215, 231
Chicago Medical College
15, 39
China 108

Chinese Restaurant Syn-
drome 202
Christopher, Frederick 96
Cincinnati, Ohio 12, 26, 216,
228
Cincinnati College 23
Cincinnati Medical College
162
Civil War 36, 57, 100, 165
Clagett, Theron 55, 78, 187
Cleveland, Ohio 25, 37, 110,
179
Cleveland Clinic 235
Cobb, Farrar 183
Coburn, Alvin 234
Codman, Ernest 232
Cole, Warren 104
College of Medicine of the
East Carolina State
University 194
College of Philadelphia (Uni-
versity of Pennsylva-
nia) 57
Coller, Frederick 182
Collier's Magazine 166
Collins, Asa 102, 145
Colorado, state of 101
Columbia, South Carolina
13, 127
Comanche, Texas 94
Command and General Staff
College 242
Coney Island, New York 104
Connecticut, state of 11, 126,
139, 154
Connecticut River Colony
154
Cook County Hospital 75,
83, 118

White, William A. 240
Wiggers, Carl 19
Williams, John 52
Williams, William Carlos 17
Winthrop, John 126, 154
Wisconsin, state of 100
Wishard, William 7
Withington, Alfreda 123
Woman's Hospital (New
  York) 14
Women's Medical College of
  Pennsylvania 117
Wooster Medical School 25
World War I 68
World War II 48
Wyeth, John 34
Wyoming, state of 146

Y

Yale University 114
Yale Medical School 138
Young, Hugh 129, 177

Errata Sheet

Chapter 3

P. 25, par.3, line 2: "William Osier" should read "William Osler."

P. 25, par.3, line 5: "Osier" should read "Osler."

P. 27, par.5, line 2: "Howard Rush" should read "Howard Rusk"

P. 28, line 1: "Dr: Rush" should read "Dr. Rusk."

P. 32, par.4, line 1: "James Newton" should read "James Mathews."

P. 32, last line: "pink other hands" should read "pink of her hands."

P. 33, line 3: "other tress" should read "of her tress."

Chapter 4

P. 47, par.3, line 1: "William Osier" should read "William Osler."

P. 47, par.3, line 11: "Osier" should read "Osler."

Chapter 6

P. 76, par.4, line 3: "Alien Street" should read "Allen Street."

P. 76, last line of the verse, "Alien Street" should read "Allen Street."

P. 76, first prose line after the verse, "Alien Street" should read "Allen Street."

Chapter 8

P. 109, par.4, line 2: "William Osier" should read "William Osler."

P. 109, par.4, line 11: "Dr. Osier" should read "Dr.Osler."

Chapter 11

P.159, par.4, line 2: "Corn huskers" should read "Cornhuskers."

P. 164, par.3, line 2: "Dr. Osier" should read "Dr. Osler."

P. 164, par.3, line 3: "And Osier" should read "And Osler."

P. 164, par.3, line 7: "Osier" should read "Osler."

Chapter 13

P. 191, par.5, line 4: should read, "told of abdomodal (abdominal) surgery, of a pindex (appendix) operation."

P. 191, par.5, line 7: "llgu blatter" should read "gull blatter."

Chapter 14

P. 214, par.2, line 2: "school" should read "schl."

P. 214, par.2, line 5: "prgrss rites" should read "prgrss ntes."

P. 214, par.5, line 4: "erroneous. The author" should read "erroneous: the author."

Chapter 16

P. 243, par.3, line 7: "American Nervousuesa" should read "American Nervousness."

Sources

Adair, Fred L. *The Country Doctor and the Specialist,* 1968.

Adams. Samuel H. "Peruna and the Bracers," *Colliers Weekly,* 28 Oct. 1905.

Albee, Fred W. A. *Surgeon's Fight to Rebuild Men,* 1943.

Albee, Louella B. *Doctor and I,* 1951.

Alter, J.C. ed. *The Journal of Priddy Meeks,* Utah Hist Q 10:145, 1942.

Andreason, Nancy C. In Trautmann, Joanne, *Healing Arts in Dialogue,* 1981.

Aub, Joseph. *Pioneer in Modern Medicine,* 1970.

Aughinbaugh, W.E. *I Swear By Apollo,* 1936.

Bailey, Charles P. In Weisse, Allen B. *Conversations in Medicine,* 1984.

Baker, Sara Josephine. *Fighting For Life,* 1939.

Barber, Laura ed. *The Doctors Herff,* 2 vols, 1973.

Barnes, Ann Brace. "Women in Medicine. The Oral History Project of the Medical College of Pennsylvania." Interview by Regina Morantz, 1977.

Barringer, Emily. *Bowery To Bellewe,* 1950.

Bartuska, Doris. *Women in Medicine,* op. cit.

Bean, William B. "The Munchausen Syndrome," Perspect Biol Med 2:347-353, 1958-59.

Berczeller, Peter H. *Doctors and Patients,* 1994.

Bergom, Ronald O. "A Small Town Hero," JAMA 261:2548, 1989.

Bernheim, Bertram. *Story of the Johns Hopkins,* 1948.

Black, John. *Forty Years in the Medical Profession,* 1900.

Blackwell, Elizabeth. *Pioneer Work in Opening the Medical Profession to Women,* 1895.

Bluestone, Naomi. *So You Want To Be a Doctor,* 1981.

Bond, Douglas D. In Cope, Oliver, *Man, Mind and Medicine,* 1968.

Bossard, Marcus. *Eighty-one Years of Living,* 1946.

Bourgeois, Stephen. In Scherr, George, *Best of the Journal of Irreproducible Results,* p59-60, 1983.

Bourne, Alec. W. *Doctor's Creed,* 1962.

Braasch, William F. *Early Days in the Mayo Clinic,* 1969.

Brasset, Edmund. *A Doctor's Pilgrimage,* 1951.

Brewer, Walpole. *Eden Clay,* 1928.

Brown, Marvin. *House Calls,* 1988.

Bruce, Nadine V. *Women in Medicine,* op. cit.

Bucy, Paul C. *Neurosurgical Giants,* 1985.

Bucy, Paul C. "A Philosophy of Neurosurgery," Clin Neurosurg 8:64-77, 1962.

Burnum, John M. "Dialect is Diagnostic," Ann Int Med 100:899-901, 1984.

Burr, Colonel Bell. *Medical History of Michigan,* 2 vols, 1930.

Byam, William. *The Road to Harley Street,* 1963.

Caleel, Richard T. *Surgeon, A Year in the Life of an Inner-City Doctor,* 1986.

Sources

Cassidy, Frederick C. *Dictionary of American Regional English,* 4 vols, 1985-2002.

Cavender, Anthony ed. *A Folk Lexicon of South Central Appalachia,* 1990.

Chaffee, John S. *Reflections on Erie County Physicians, Private,* 1990.

Christopher, Frederick. *One Surgeon's Practice,* 1957.

Clagett, O. Theron. *Reflections,* 1979.

Cobb, Farrar. *Boston Surgeon,* 1986.

Coburn, Alvin F. *Commitment Total,* 1974.

Codman, Ernest A. *The Shoulder,* 1934.

Coe, Edith. *Hertzler Heritage,* 1975.

Collins, Asa W. *Doctor Asa,* 1941.

Connaughton, Dennis. *Warren Cole M.D. and the Ascent of Scientific Surgery,* 1991.

Corea, Gena. "Dorothy Reed Mendenhall," Ms Magazine, April, 1974.

Corner, George. *The Seven Ages of a Medical Scientist,* 1981.

Cosens, William B. *Your Servant the Doctor,* 1931:

Crile, George. *An Autobiography,* 2 vols. 1947.

Cunningham, John. *As the Twig is Bent,* 1936.

DaCosta, John C. *The Trials and Triumphs of the Surgeon,* ed. Frederick C. Keller, 1944.

DaCosta, John C. Selections From Papers and Speeches, 1931

Davidoff, Leo M. *A Tree Not For Myself,* 1975.

Davis, Audry. W. *Dr. Kelly of Hopkins,* 1959.

Davis, Loyal. *A Surgeon's Odyssey,* 1973.

Davis, Minney. "Mary Elizabeth Bates," Med Woman's J 55:30-31,1948.

de Savitsch, Eugene. *In Search of Complications,* 1940.

Despelder, L.A. and Strickland, A.L. *Last Dance,* 1944.

Diller, Theodore. *Pioneer Medicine in Western Pennsylvania,* 1927.

Dirckx, John H. Doctor, "I'm [sic]," Am J Dermatopathol 14:369-371, 1992.

Dolby, Karen. *Women in Medicine,* op.cit.

Dole, Mary P. *A Doctor in Homespun,* 1941.

Doyle, Helen MasKnight. *A Child Went Forth,* 1934:

Dockerty, Malcom B. Rhymed *Reminiscences of a Pathologist,* 1980.

Douglas, James. *Journal and Reminiscences,* 1910.

Dragstedt, Carl A. "Verse after," Perspect Biol Med 14:172, 1970-71.

Drake, Daniel. *Practical Essays on Education and the Medical Profession in the United States,* 1832.

Drake, Daniel. *Pioneer Life in Kentucky,* ed. Drake, Charles D., 1870.

Drooz Ircna Gross. *Doctor of Medicine,* 1949.

Dugan, Daniel O. "Laughter & Tears: Best Medicine For Stress," Nursing Forum 24:18-26,1989.

Earnest, Ernst. *P. S. Weir Mitchell,* 1950.

Sources

Evans, William. *Journey to Harley Street, 1968.* Fabricant, Noah. *Why We Became Doctors,* 1954.

Fearn, Ann Walter. *My Days of Strength,* 1939.

Finland, Maxwell & Castle, *Wm. B. Comps. The Harvard Medical Unit at Boston City Hospital,* 1982.

Finney, John M.T.A. *A Surgeon's Life,* 1940.

Fisher, James & Hawley, Lowell S. *A Few Buttons Missing,* 1951.

Fleming, David. In Konner, Melvin, op. cit. p21

Fleming, Donald. *William H Welch and the Rise of Modern Medicine,* 1954.

Fox, George. *Reminiscences,* 1926.

Fox, Corey. In Ellenbogan, Glenn S. *Oral Sadism and the Vegetarian Personality,* 1987.

Furman, Richard. *To Be a Surgeon,* 1982.

Gibbs, Samuel E. "The Influence of Trifles," Medical Pickwick 8:364-367,1922.

Gibbs, Samuel E. Leaves "From an Old Notebook," Medical Life 29:558-567,1922.

Gifford, Edward S. *Father Against the Devil,* 1966.

Golden, Francis L. *What the Doctor Ordered,* 1949.

Gordon, Benjamin. *Between Two Worlds,* 1952.

Gordon, Maurice. *Aesculapius Comes to the Colonies,* 1949.

Greben, Stanley. *Love's Labor,* 1985.

Gross, Samuel. *Autobiography,* 1887.

Hall, Edward. "Reminiscences of Dr. John Park," American Antiquarian Society Proc. 7:69-93,1890.

Hamilton, Alexander. *Gentleman's Progress,* ed. Carl Bridenbaugh, reprint ed. 1948.

Hardy, Harriet L. *Challenging Man-Made Diseases,* 1983.

Harrison, Michelle. *A Woman in Residence,* 1983.

Harvey, A. McGehee. "John Whitridge Williams," Johns Hopkins Med J 138:96-101,1976.

Henry, Frederick P. *Standard History of the Medical Profession of Philadelphia,* 1897.

Herman, Leon. *A Surgeon Thinks it Over,* 1962

Hertzler, Arthur. *Horse and Buggy Doctor,* 1938.

Hessel, Susan. "The Gundersen Legacy," Harv Med Alumni Bull 65:42-48,(Winter) 1991-92.

Holmes, Oliver Wendell. *Medical Essays,* 1861

Homans, John. "Reminiscences," Harv Med Alumni Bull 24:103-111 (June) 1950.

Hood, Tom. "(From, Whims and Oddities)" St. Bartholomews Hosp J 21:116, 1913-1914.

Hopkinson, Francis. *Miscellaneous Essays & Occasional Writings,* 1792.

Hutchison, Robert. In Scarlett, E.P., "Table Talk," Arch Int Med 114:843-849,1964.

Irving, Frederick C. *Safe Deliverance,* 1942.

Sources

Jackson, Chevalier. *The Life of Chevalier Jackson,* 1938.

Jerger, Joseph. *Doctor -Here's Your Hat,* 1939.

Johnson, Charles B, *Sixty Years in Msdisal Harness;* 1928.

Johnson, Edith. *Leaves From a Doctor's Diary,* 1954.

Juettner, Otto. *Daniel Drake and His Followers,* 1909.

Kahn, Edgar A. *Journal of a Neurosurgeon,* 1972.

Keen, W. W. *Memoirs of William Williams Keen,* ed. James, W. W.Keen, 1990.

Kellogg, David S. *A Doctor at All Hours,* ed. Everest, Allan S, 1970.

Kessler, Henry. *The Knife is Not Enough,* 1968.

Kimmelstiel, Ruth. *In Finland & Castle,* op. cit. vol. 2 ,Pt.2.

King, George S. *Doctor on a Bicycle,* 1958.

Kinney, Janet. *Saga of a Surgeon,* 1987.

Kolin, Philip. "The Language of Nursing," American Speech, 48:192-210, 1973.

Konner, Melvin. *Becoming a Doctor,* 1987.

Landers, Ann. Syndicated newspaper column, 12 July, 1992.

Lawson, Lewis. "Walker Percy's Physicians and Patients," Literature and Medicine,3:130-141,1984.

Leaf, Alexander. "After Carl Popper," p108 Proc Assoc Am Physicians 108:107-109,1996.

Leonard, Arnold A. Chief, *Owen Wangensteen Festschrift,* 1967.

Lillard, John F. *The Medical Muse,* 1896.

Loomis, Frederick. *Consultation Room,* 1939.

Lovejoy, "Esther Clayson." Oreg Hist Q 75:7-36,1974.

Lyons, John B. *William Henry Drummond: Poet in Patois,* 1994.

Macartney, William N. *Fifty Years a Country Doctor,* 1938.

Macdonald, Greville. *Reminiscences of a Specialist,* 1932.

Magee, Joni. In Morantz, Regina et. al., op.cit.

Manley, Woods H. *The Doctor's Wyoming Children,* 1953.

Manuel, Barry M. "A Contemporary Physician's Oath," New Eng J Med 318:521-22, 1988.

Martin, Franklin. *The Joy of Living,* 1933.

Martin, Toni. *How to Survive Medical School,* 1983.

Mason, Andrew V. *Surgeon's Log,* 1980.

Mather, Cotton. *Angel of Bethesda,* ed. Jones, Gordon, 1972.

Mather, Cotton. "In Paterna," a manuscript autobiography quoted by Beall, Otho T and Shryock, R.H. in, Cotton Mather., 1954.

Mathews, James. *The Lute of Life,* ed. Hurt,Walter, 1911.

Mayo, Charles W. *The Story of My Family,* 1968.

Mayo,Charles W. "Something About My Father," Mayo Clin Proc 64:707-714, 1989.

McNair, Rush. *Medical Memoirs of 50 Years in Kalamazoo,* 1936.

Medical Pickwick. "A Unique Tombstone" 1:160, 1915.

Medved,Michael. *Hospital,* 1982.

Meigs,Charles D. "Biographical Notice of Daniel Drake M.D.," Trans Coll Physicians Phila 2:6-41,1853-6

Michner, Ezra. *Autobiographical Notes,* 1893.

Sources

Middleton, George W. *Memoirs of a Pioneer Surgeon,* 1976.

Middleton, Wm. S. "Joseph Leidy, Scientist," Ann Med Hist 5:100-112, 1923.

Moore, G.A. In Moulton,Charles W. ed. "Doctor's Leisure Hour" 10:300. Moorman, Lewis J. Pioneer Doctor, 1951.

Morantz, Regina M. et. al. *In Her Own Words,* 1982.

Morgan, Kenneth. *A Little Stork Told Me,* 1966.

Moms, Robert T. *Doctors Versus Folks,* 1915.

Morse, John T. *The Works of Oliver Wendell Holmes,* 15 vols. 1896.

Morse, John T. *The Life and Letters of Oliver Wendell Holmes,* 2 vols. 1896.

Morton, Rosalie *Slaughter. A Woman Surgeon,* 1937.

Morton, Thomas G. *The History of the Pennsylvania Hospital,* 1937.

Mosher, Eliza. *New York Times,* 29 March 1925, Sect 9, p5.

Nelson, Douglas S. "Humor in a Pediatric Emergency Department," Pediatrics 89:1089-1092,1992.

Nixon, Pat I. *The Medical Story of Early Texas,* 1946.

Nolen, William A. *The Making of a Surgeon,* 1970.

"Ode to the Skeleton." See Can J Med Surg 19:224, 1906.

O'Toole,K. et. al. "Removing Cockroaches From the Auditory Canal," New Eng J Med 312:1197, 1985.

Parker, Beulah. *Evolution of a Psychiatrist,* 1987.

Pickard, Madge & Buley, R.C. *The Midwest Pioneer,* 1945.

Pound, Louise. "American Euphemisms For Dying, Death and Burial," American Speech 11:195-202,1936.

Pusey, William A. *A Doctor of the 1870s,* 1932.

Pyle, Eleanor. "Fuller Albright's Inimitable Style," Harv Mod Alumni Bull 56:46-51 (Fall), 1982.

Raffensperger, John ed. *The Old Lady on Harrison Street,* 1997.

Reddall, Henry F. *Wit and Humor of the Physician,* 1906.

Redman, Jack C. "A Wet Mouse," JAMA 252:901,1984.

Rehwinkel, Alfred & Efner, Bessie L. *Dr. Bessie,*1963.

Reifler, Douglas R. "Special Delivery," JAMA 262:96, 1989

Reilly, Philip. *To Do No Harm,* 1987.

Rivers, Thomas M. *Reflections on a Life in Medicine and Science,* ed. Benison, Saul, 1967.

Robinson, James O. *Frederick A. Coller,* 1987.

Robinson, Judith. *Tom Cullen of Baltimore,* 1944.

Rooker, James I. "Thirty-three Years a Country Doctor," Trans Indiana St Med Soc 121-128, 1889.

Rosen, Samuel. *Autobiography of Dr. Samuel Rosen,* 1973.

Rosser, Charles M. *Doctors and Doctors,* 1941.

Rush, Benjamin. *Letters of Benjamin Rush,* ed. Butterfield, Lyman H., 1951

Rush, Benjamin. In Corner, George ed. *The Autobiography of Benjamin Rush,* 1948.

Rusk, Howard. *A World To Care For,* 1972.

Sources

Scarlett, E.P. "Some Hoaxes in Medical History and Literature," ArchInt Med 113:291-296,1964.

Scarlett, E.P. As cited after Hutchison, prayer beginning"Lord, Thou knowest.." attributed to the Southwark Diocese Magazine, London, England, n.d.,n.p.

Scheie, Harold D. Ophthalmology Oral History Series. Interview by Sally Hughes, 1988.

Schmidt, Jacob E. *Dictionary of Medical Slang,* 1959.

Schreiber, Frederick C. "Surgical Gambits," Harper Hosp Bull 17:314-21, 1959.

SchcVartz; Stanley, N. "Medcl Spdwriting," New Eng J Med 321:764-765, 1989.

Scott, Margaret H. *Say "Ah",* 1981.

Sharpe, William. *Brain Surgeon,* 1952.

Shatuck, George. *A Memoir of Frederick Cheever Shatuck,* 1967.

Shorter, Edward. *Bedside Manners,* 1985.

Sims, J. Marion. *The Story of My Life,* 1884.

Sirridge, Marjorie. *Women in Medicine,* op. cit.

Sloop, Mary T. Martin. *Miracle in the Hills,* 1953.

Snyder, Richard W. et. al. "Mediastinal Emphysema After a Sax Orgy," New Eng J Med 323:758, 1990.

Speer, Robert I. "The Incredible George Morris Gray," J Kansas Med Soc 66:142-146,1965.

Spiegel, Ann. *Women in Medicine,* op. cit.

Stanley, G.D. "Medical Pioneering in Alberta," HiSt Bull, 11;57-63,1946.

Starzl, Thomas E. *The Puzzle People,* 1992.

Stead, Eugene. *What This Patient Needs is a Doctor,* 1978.

Stearns, Carl M. (re John W. Coolidge) *Early History of Medicine in Sullivan County,NH,* 1974.

Stewart, Margaret. *From Dugout to Hilltop,* 1951:

Stitt, Pauline. *Women in Medicine,,* op. cit.

Stitt, Pauline. In Morantz, Regina, et. al. op. cit.

Stone, Mildred. *Hen Medic,* 1989.

Stratton, Owen T. *Medicine Man,* 1989.

Strauss, Maurice B. *Familiar Medical Quotations,* 1968.

Szasz, Thomas S. *A Lexicon of Lunacy,* 1933.

Talbott, John A and Manevitz, Alan Z.A. eds. *Psychiatric House Calls,* 1988.

Taylor, Harvey G. *Rememberances and Reflections,* 1991.

Thomas, Lewis. *The Youngest Science,* 1983

Thoms,Herbert. *Jared Eliot, Minister, Doctor, Scientist and His Connecticut,* 1967.

Thorns, Herbert. *The Heritage of Connecticut Medicine,* 1942.

Thompson, Elizabeth. *Harvey Cushing,* 1981.

Tomkins, Pendleton. "Recollections of Charles Frazier," Trans Stud Coll Physicians Phila S5, 12:491-497, 1990.

Sources

Trowbridge, Eunice & Radbill, April. *Dr. Josephine Evarts, A Tribute,* 1981.

Van Hoosen, Bertha. *Petticoat Surgeon,* 1947.

Vaughan, Victor C. *A Doctor's Memories,* 1926.

Warren, John Collins, "Reminiscences," Md Med J 44:45-54 1901.

Warren, John C. *To Work in the Vineyards of Surgery,* ed. Churchill, Edward D., 1958.

Waisgii, Allorl, *Conversations in Medicine,* 1984,

Welch, Claude E. *A Twentieth Century Surgeon,* 1992.

Welch, Claude E. "A Student Becomes a Surgeon," JAMA 259:3168-1988.

Welch, Lillian. *Reminiscences of Thirty Years in Baltimore,* 1925.

Welch, William J. *What Happened in Between,* 1972.

Weston, William. "Memories of a Busy Life," S Carolina Med Assoc J 56:269-276, 1960.

Wheeler, John B. Menpoirs of a Small Town Surgeon, 1935.

White, Benjamin. V. *Stanley Cobb,* 1984.

White, William A. *The Autobiography of a Purpose,* 1938.

Wiggers, Carl. J. *Reminiscences and Adventures in Circulation Research,* 1958.

Wild, John & Harkey, Ira. *Alton Ochsner, Surgeon of the South,* 1990.

Wishard, Elizabeth M. *A Doctor of the Old School,* 1920.

Withington, Alfreda. *Mine Eyes Have Seen,* 1941.

Wolf, Marguerite. *How to be a Doctor's Wife Without Really Dying,* 1978.

Wyeth, John A. *With Sabre and Scalpel,* 1914.

Young, Hugh H. *A Surgeon's Autobiography,* 1940.

Zahorsky, John. *From the Hills,* 1949.

Zakrzewska, Maria. *A Woman's Quest,* ed. Victor; Agnes C., 1924.

Acknowledgments:
The Human Nature Chart is reprinted with permission from Medical Economics, May 1934.